AF572625

Diagnostic Ultrasound in Gastrointestinal Disease

CLINICS IN DIAGNOSTIC ULTRASOUND
VOLUME 1

Forthcoming Volumes in the Series

Vol. 2 Genitourinary Ultrasonography, Arthur T. Rosenfield, Guest Editor

Vol. 3 Diagnostic Ultrasound in Obstetrics, John C. Hobbins, Guest Editor

Vol. 4 Diagnostic Ultrasound in Cardiology, Joseph A. Kisslo, Guest Editor

Vol. 5 New Techniques and Instrumentation, P. N. T. Wells, Guest Editor

Vol. 6 Diagnostic Ultrasound in Endocrinology, W. F. Sample, Guest Editor

Diagnostic Ultrasound in Gastrointestinal Disease

Edited by

Kenneth J. W. Taylor, M.D., Ph.D.

Associate Professor
Department of Diagnostic Radiology
Yale University School of Medicine
New Haven, Connecticut

CHURCHILL LIVINGSTONE

NEW YORK, EDINBURGH AND LONDON 1979

CHURCHILL LIVINGSTONE
Medical Division of Longman Inc.

Distributed in the United Kingdom by Churchill Livingstone, 23 Ravelston Terrace, Edinburgh EH4 3TL and by associated companies, branches and representatives throughout the world.

First published 1979

ISBN 0 443 08046 1

Library of Congress Cataloging in Publication Data
Main entry under title:

Diagnostic ultrasound in gastrointestinal disease.

(Clinics in diagnostic ultrasound; v. 1)
1. Digestive organs—Diseases—Diagnosis.
2. Diagnosis, Ultrasonic. I. Taylor, Kenneth J. W., 1939– II. Series. [DNLM: 1. Ultrasonics—Diagnostic use. 2. Gastrointestinal diseases—Diagnosis. WI141 D534]
RC804.U4D5 616.3′07′54 78-21895
ISBN 0–443–08046–1

Printed in USA

Contributors

Orla Als, M.D.
Department of Urology, Ultrasonic Laboratory, Herlev Hospital, University of Copenhagen, Denmark

Jason Cordell Birnholz, M.D.
Assistant Professor of Radiology, Harvard Medical School; Radiologist-in-Chief, Boston Hospital for Women; Director, Clinical Ultrasound, Peter Bent Brigham Hospital; Adv. Academic Fellow, James Picker Foundation, Boston, Massachusetts

David Cosgrove, M.A., M.Sc., M.R.C.P.
Consultant in Nuclear Medicine & Ultrasound, Royal Marsden Hospital, London, England

Michael Crade, M.D.
Instructor in Diagnostic Radiology, Yale University School of Medicine, New Haven, Connecticut

Casper S. de Graaff, M.D.
Department of Internal Medicine, Groningen University, Groningen, The Netherlands

Alan G. Dembner, M.D.
Attending Radiologist; Chief of Diagnostic Ultrasound, St. Barnabas Medical Center, Livingston, New Jersey

Jens Gammelgaard, M.D.
Research Associate, Ultrasonic Laboratory, Herlev Hospital, University of Copenhagen, Denmark

Fred Gorelick, M.D.
Fellow in Gastroenterology, Yale University School of Medicine, New Haven, Connecticut

Hans Henrik Holm, M.D.
Chief Surgeon, Head of Ultrasound Unit, Herlev Hospital, University of Copenhagen, Denmark

Janet E. Husband, M.R.C.P., F.R.C.R.
Research Fellow in Diagnostic Radiology and Honorary Senior Lecturer, Institute of Cancer Research, The Royal Marsden Hospital, Sutton, England

Hylton B. Meire, M.B., B.S., F.R.C.R.
Consultant in Ultrasound, Clinical Research Center, Harrow, England

Arthur T. Rosenfield, M.D.
Associate Professor of Diagnostic Radiology, Yale University School of Medicine; Attending Radiologist, Yale–New Haven Hospital, New Haven, Connecticut

W. Frederick Sample, M.D.
Associate Professor of Radiology; Co-Director, Section of Ultrasound and Computed Body Tomography, UCLA School of Medicine, Los Angeles, California

Dennis A. Sarti, M.D.
Assistant Professor of Radiology; Co-Director, Section of Ultrasound and Computed Body Tomography, UCLA School of Medicine, Los Angeles, California

Joseph F. Simeone, M.D.
Assistant Professor of Diagnostic Radiology, Harvard Medical School; Assistant in Radiology, Massachusetts General Hospital, Boston, Massachusetts

Bruce D. Simonds, M.D.
Assistant Clinical Professor, Department of Diagnostic Radiology; Attending Physician, Yale University, New Haven, Connecticut

Howard M. Spiro, M.D.
Professor of Medicine; Chief, Gastrointestinal Section, Yale University School of Medicine, New Haven, Connecticut

William B. Steel, M.D.
Assistant Chief, Department of Radiology; Director, Division of Ultrasound, Hutzel Hospital, Detroit Medical Center, Detroit, Michigan

Daniel Sullivan, M.D.
Assistant Professor of Radiology, Duke University Medical Center, Durham, North Carolina

Kenneth J. W. Taylor, M.D., Ph.D.
Associate Professor of Radiology, Yale–New Haven Hospital, New Haven, Connecticut

Contents

CASE REPORTS

Foreword

With the rapid proliferation in the number of books, one can indeed question the need for yet another. However, ultrasound is a new subject and there are at present very few journals devoted to it. Furthermore, the subject is changing rapidly and long delays await any article to be published in the radiological literature, so that published articles lag far behind current thought. Review articles tend to be even more out-dated, since they review the original literature from time to time and are themselves subjected to rewriting and publishing delays. We therefore believe that there is a need for authoritative review articles from centers that are very active in ultrasound, which will reflect contemporary thought on this rapidly changing subject.

It is the intention of this series to devote each issue to one subject, each organized by a Guest Editor. For the first few issues, these editors will be the members of the Editorial Board, who will produce the following further titles:

1979 Genitourinary Ultrasonography—Arthur T. Rosenfield, M.D.
Diagnostic Ultrasound in Obstetrics—John Hobbins, M.D.

1980 Diagnostic Ultrasound in Cardiology—Joseph Kisslo, M.D.
New Techniques and Instrumentation in Diagnostic Ultrasound—Peter N.T. Wells, Ph.D.
Diagnostic Ultrasound in Endocrinology—Frederick Sample, M.D.

Each editor will invite authors of acknowledged expertise to review a given subject, providing approximately ten articles per issue. It is hoped that this will summarize contemporary thought for the practicing radiologist as it pertains to the state-of-the-art in ultrasound techniques.

This first issue of the Clinics in Diagnostic Ultrasound is on Gastroenterology. It is hoped that this issue will be of interest not only to radiologists, but also to referring physicians in gastroenterology and internal medicine. It is important for the radiologist to appreciate the clinical problems involved in therapeutic decisions, so we invited the staff of our gastrointestinal unit, including its Chief, Dr. Howard Spiro, to contribute to this issue on the indications and efficacy of ultrasound examination from the clinician's viewpoint. We believe that this will be a valuable addition to the contributions from radiologists.

In this issue we have attempted to cover the entire field of gastroenterology to which ultrasound can make an important contribution at the present state of its development. The contributors include ultrasonologists from both east and west coasts of the United States, the United Kingdom and Denmark. We believe that the opinions expressed in each of these contributions reflect the state-of-the-art.

Finally, we have arranged a self-evaluation section in which clinical problems are presented together with the ultrasound examinations, and the solutions discussed on the reverse page. It is hoped that this will present the reader with an opportunity to assess objectively what he has learned from the perusal of this issue. We welcome constructive criticism of this format and hope that these periodic reviews on diagnostic ultrasound will prove to be a valuable learning experience for their readers.

Kenneth J. W. Taylor

The Gastroenterologist's View of the Indications and Efficacy of Ultrasound Examination

FRED S. GORELICK
HOWARD M. SPIRO

The gastroenterologist, like any other subspecialist, has to choose efficiently from an increasing number of diagnostic modalities while observing economy in patient care. How this dilemma can be solved remains uncertain, but here we will consider ultrasonography from the standpoint of the concerned clinician anxious to learn and willing to appreciate aesthetics, but mainly concerned with how ultrasound can change diagnostic opinion or therapeutic approach. Generally, ultrasound seems to be an advance which is safe, of modest cost, and with broad applicability, particularly in the detection of cystic lesions within the abdomen and in the delineation of enlarged bile ducts and gallstones.

Like many new diagnostic tests, ultrasound can be used 1) to confirm a strong clinical impression or to answer a specific question, 2) to resolve ambiguity raised by other morphological studies, 3) as a broad screening test, or 4) in the follow-up of previously identified lesions. In any new diagnostic study, especially one which depends upon the skill of an observer and upon a rapidly changing technology, exact percentages are not very meaningful. Figures at one hospital may be different from those at another, partly because of the interest and experience of the observer and partly because of the different kinds of patients studied. The ultimate place of ultrasound in clinical gastroenterology remains for definition, but just as Sisyphus could not roll the stone all the way up the hill, improvements in ultrasonic technology render each year's opinion very quickly archaic. In what follows, the importance of these variables is implicit, but we will discuss the current clinical application of ultrasound and its contribution to clinical problems, recognizing overlap in the subdivisions which follow.

To Confirm A Strong Clinical Impression

The most valuable use of ultrasound at present seems to be to confirm what is already suspected or to answer a specific clinical question.

Pancreatic Disease

Carcinoma of the pancreas

Pancreatic carcinoma stands as the model disorder in which ultrasound can confirm the clinical impression. DiMagno et al[1] reviewed 70 patients suspected of having pancreatic carcinoma, in 30 of whom the diagnosis was confirmed at operation. Ultrasound was used to determine whether the pancreas was diseased, a specific diagnosis of pancreatic cancer not being required in this study. Only 75 percent of the patients who eventually proved to have *any* kind of pancreatic disease, including cancer or pancreatitis, were identified by ultrasound, a figure disappointing to the optimistic diagnostician. Moreover, about 30 percent of patients with cancer were already jaundiced; in the jaundiced patient the clinician can always opt for laparotomy so that a diagnosis of pancreatic disease in a patient with jaundice who still requires operation does not represent a significant diagnostic triumph. The paper did not provide information on how well ultrasound furthered the diagnosis in patients who were not jaundiced, nor how many patients had such overt disease at the time of study that ultrasound, though diagnostically correct, was not really clinically useful.

These are the kinds of questions that are never asked in the early enthusiasm for any new diagnostic technology; but they are worth evaluating early, for their answers are what the clinician needs for his diagnostic choices. The specific percentages at this stage are unimportant, although it is disappointing that Levitt et al[2] correctly identified by ultrasound only 60 percent of patients with pancreatic carcinoma, and Husband et al[3] identified only five out of nine patients. As we have already pointed out, advances in technology will no doubt raise the percentage of correct diagnoses, but still the clinician will watch to see how small a lesion will be detected by ultrasound and whether a minimal lesion can be detected before metastases have occurred. Most important of all, he will want to know whether ultrasound can ever distinguish pancreatic carcinoma from an inflammatory mass. He may regard the demonstration by ultrasound of a pancreatic mass in a 60 year old man with diabetes, weight loss, and unrelenting abdominal pain as no more helpful than the contrast studies which now show a different facet of the same mass. That McCormack et al[4] could show no increased survival after ultrasound diagnosis of pancreatic cancer underlines the clinical problem—symptoms which lead to any investigation usually come too late for therapy to help. However much the sensitivity of ultrasound improves, its benefits may be limited by the late onset of symptoms. The most that the clinician can hope for is that ultrasound will shorten the time to diagnosis and make the diagnostic approach easier for patient and clinician.

For the latter, ultrasound may prove the greatest help in guiding biopsy needles to pancreatic masses. Hancke et al[5] and Smith et al[6] each demonstrated the safety and accuracy of percutaneous pancreatic biopsy, and the procedure is being more widely adopted. Pancreatic biopsy may not affect survival, but in the patient who is not jaundiced, it may make chemotherapy and irradiation possible without the need for exploration. So far, however, such diagnostic confirmation depends upon the keen eye of the cytopathologist.

It has even been suggested that different types of pancreatic tumors, carcinoma and lymphoma for example, may reflect diagnostic echogenic patterns because of varying cellular composition, density, pattern of invasion, and desmoplastic response. Only 100 percent reliability would give real help in this regard without biopsy. As the pancreas is the second commonest site of intraabdominal lymphoma, such echographic distinctions would indeed be very helpful. A few patients with gastrinomas have been reported in whom no neoplasm was identified by ultrasound or CT scan; a very small tumor or one with cells not so different from those of the parent organ may not be readily detected by ultrasound.

Pancreatic pseudocyst

It is in the demonstration of pancreatic pseudocysts that ultrasound has proven such an enormous boon. Before ultrasound, documentation of a pseudocyst was difficult, requiring indirect evidence of presence and size by barium studies, arteriography, or endoscopic pancreatography. Pancreatic pseudocysts are now distinguished with ease from the pancreatic phlegmon which in the past provided such a problem in differential diagnosis for the clinician. With its definitive and noninvasive depiction of a pseudocyst, ultrasound has made other techniques generally obsolete for diagnosis and follow-up. Ultrasound has reminded the clinician that a pseudocyst may be present with minimal or no enzymatic abnormalities, that they are more common than previously suspected, and may resolve spontaneously. How small a pseudocyst can be detected and its clinical significance remain subjects for study however, as pathologists have long found incidental pseudocysts at autopsy. Doust and Pearce[7] detected cysts as small as one centimeter, but also failed to demonstrate a one centimeter pseudocyst in the tail of the pancreas later seen at endoscopic pancreatography. Kressel et al[8] compared CT scans with ultrasound in the diagnosis of surgically proven pseudocysts and reported that ultrasound found a pseudocyst in seven of eight patients but, because of extensive bowel gas, missed two of four with infected pseudocysts. The following is an example of a patient with a pseudocyst we have followed.

> A 29 year-old male chronic alcoholic with a 3 year history of recurrent bouts of pancreatitis, was admitted with pain, nausea and vomiting. On physical examination, he had hepatomegaly, but no other evidence of chronic liver disease. There was a tender area of increased fullness in the right upper quadrant. The serum amylase was slightly elevated at 183 (nl<155) with a normal serum lipase An abdominal X-ray revealed a few calcifications at the head of the pancreas. An abdominal ultrasound examination at this time revealed a large pseudocyst of the pancreas (Figure 1a and b). The patient was treated conservatively and did well. Six weeks later, repeat ultrasound demonstrated some diminution in the size of the pseudocyst (Figure 1c and d). A third examination (Figure 1e and f) four months later, when the patient was asymptomatic and the mass no longer palpable, documented disappearance of the pseudocyst, although the remaining pancreatic echogenic abnormalities were suggestive of residual pancreatic disease.

This case illustrates what we now appreciate as one of the natural histories of the pancreatic pseudocyst. We need to know more from prospective studies relating sonographic findings to clinical course. Do smaller pseudocysts have a greater probability of resolving or a lesser chance of becoming infected? How soon in the course of pancreatitis does a pseudocyst form, and does its location in the gland affect the possibility of spontaneous drainage?

Acute pancreatitis

Ultrasound should be helpful in the patient with pancreatitis not only to exclude gallstones, but also to confirm an uncertain diagnosis or to look for a pseudocyst in the patient with recurrent or protracted disease. Ileus, so characteristic of pancreatitis, may limit the contribution of ultrasound by making satisfactory examination of the pancreas difficult in the acute stages. In a retrospective study, the overall accuracy in the diagnosis of acute pancreatitis was about 80 percent, but the 16 percent of normal controls who also had an "enlarged pancreas" suggests an uncomfortable degree of overlap.[7] A similar degree of accuracy has been reported by Husband et al.[3] Following 12 patients with acute pancreatitis, Doust and Pearce[7] reported that serum enzyme levels usually return to normal before echographic resolution, a sequence similar to that already recognized in pancreatitis, with the rapid fall of amylase levels to normal despite continuing clinical manifestations.

Evidence of biliary tract disease in patients with acute pancreatitis is the most helpful evidence of all. The demonstration of gallstones in patients with acute pancreatitis is particularly helpful but, to the clinician, demonstration of dilated biliary ducts on ultrasound may mean obstruction either by stones in the common duct or simply by inflammation in the head of the pancreas. In an appropriate clinical setting, ultrasound may well prove diagnostic of pancreatitis, but no doubt it will not replace the simpler measurements of serum enzymes for diagnosis. Ultrasound may prove to be a guide to the seriousness of the disorder, however. The clinician will be interested in knowing whether the patient with elevated pancreatic enzymes and a normal pancreas at ultrasound has less severe disease than a patient with an abnormal pancreas at ultrasound; whether such distinctions can serve as a guide to

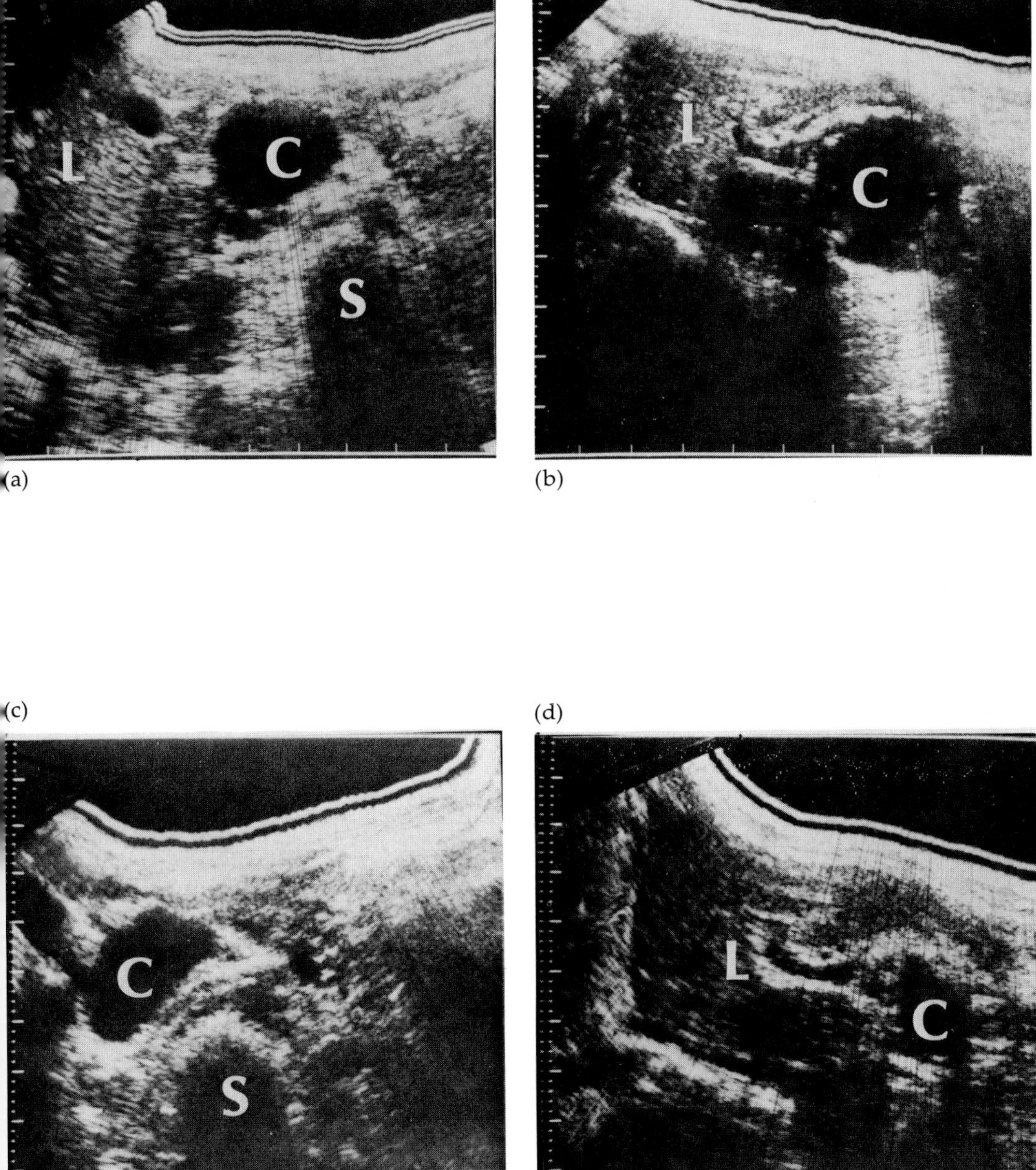

FIGURE 1. Initial ultrasound scans showing (a) transverse and (b) longitudinal views of the large pseudocyst. The second examination demonstrated some decrease in size of the pseudocyst in the (c) transverse and (d) longitudinal projection. (C = pseudocyst; L = liver; S = spine; I = inferior vena cava; P = pancreas.)

Figure 1 *continued overpage:*

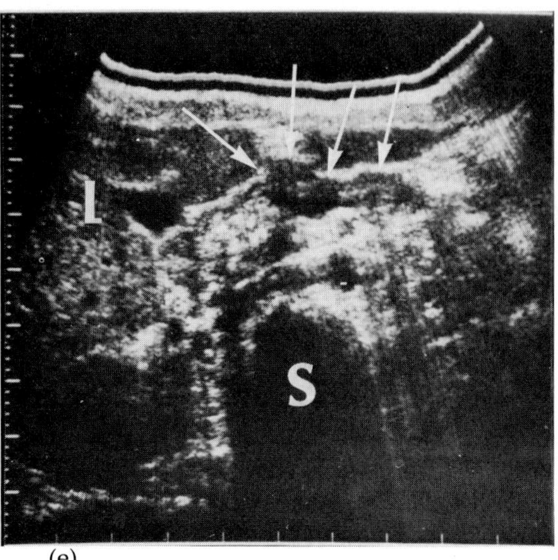

(e)

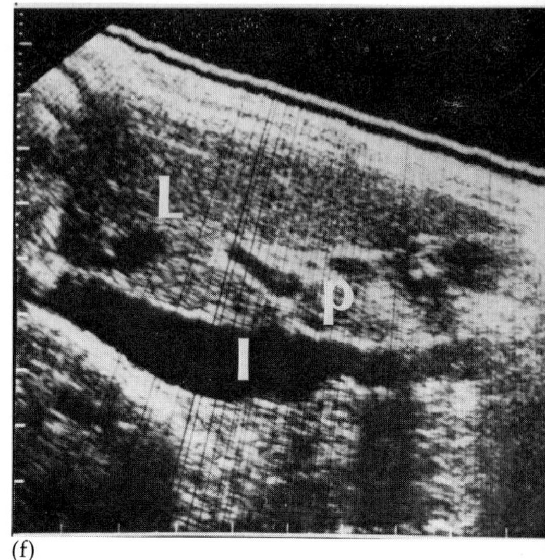

(f)

FIGURE 1 *continued.*
The final examination showed no pseudocyst, but an echogenically abnormal pancreas: (e) transverse scan (white arrows to pancreas); and (f) longitudinal scan. (C = pseudocyst; L = liver; S = spine; I = inferior vena cava; P = pancreas.)

therapy or give some idea of the severity of the process; whether a distinction can be made between interstitial pancreatitis and hemorrhagic pancreatitis; and finally how early ultrasound can detect peritoneal complications from the seepage of pancreatic enzymes. Prospective studies are indicated.

In the patient with acute pancreatitis we now get an ultrasound examination as soon as possible to exclude the possibility of gallstones. If gallstones are found, we urge early surgery for the patient who does not quickly recover. If the ultrasound is negative or technically inadequate because of intestinal gas, we usually ask for an intravenous cholangiogram to exclude the possibility of gallstones. In the patient with protracted pancreatitis, ultrasound can detect a pseudocyst and is our first diagnostic choice, but if it is not helpful, we turn to endoscopic pancreatography or CT scans. Occasionally, endoscopic pancreatography will be necessary to distinguish pseudocysts from an extraordinarily enlarged pancreatic duct. At present, we believe ultrasound to be the most useful technique for the diagnosis of pancreatic pseudocysts and for their follow-up.

Chronic pancreatitis

The detection of sonographic abnormalities in the patient with chronic pancreatitis has proven little help so far except in the detection of pseudocysts. Prominent echo-dense abnormalities in patients with chronic pancreatitis and pancreatic calcification have been reported[3], but Doust and Pearce[7] found no distinguishing characteristics except for pseudocysts in 10 of 12 patients with chronic pancreatitis. Indeed, two patients with pancreatic calcification on plain film showed normal appearances at ultrasound. Improved technology may change matters, but at present ultrasound cannot help much in the patient with chronic pancreatitis, especially as the diagnosis is usually so obvious in the alcoholic with pancreatic calcification on abdominal films.

Hepatic Disease

In the investigation of liver disease, ultrasound can evaluate 1) focal process, usually metastases or abscesses; 2) the liver parenchyma; and 3) extrahepatic changes associated with liver disease. Evaluation of focal processes will be discussed in a later section (pp. 35–58).

Diffuse liver disease

The ability of ultrasound to detect diffuse liver disease such as fat or cirrhosis may reduce the incidence of sampling error on liver biopsy, provide an indication for biopsy, and guide the needle to the right site. In an ongoing study, now at 53 patients, we have compared hepatic ultrasound with liver biopsy for evaluating the hepatic parenchyma. So far the study suggests that ultrasound can establish the relative normality of the liver and distinguish metastases from fat or fibrosis, but that moderate amounts of fat or cirrhosis are more reliably detected by liver biopsy. Although ultrasound can readily detect major amounts of fat or fibrosis, it does not reliably distinguish moderate amounts of one from the other, or either from a completely normal liver. Needle biopsy is a more sensitive, although more invasive, technique. In the ordinary alcoholic with acute "alcoholic hepatitis," the clinician may some day come to depend upon ultrasound to assess overall changes in the liver, but at present he will probably still rely on liver biopsy. There may well be times when all that is needed is to distinguish major amounts of fat or fibrosis from a normal liver, and in such circumstances the patient may be grateful for ultrasound rather than for liver biopsy. Our study confirms the impressive ability of ultrasound to detect focal lesions in the liver: in two patients, neoplasia was easily distinguished from the surrounding cirrhotic tissue, something not easily accomplished by other means. Eighteen patients with apparent metastatic disease on ultrasound had histologically proven tumor.

Extrahepatic abnormalities suggestive of liver disease

Ultrasound has some place in the detection of extrahepatic abnormalities of liver disease, to provide objective data in patients with suspected cirrhosis or confirmatory data in patients with known cirrhosis. Ultrasound has been used to assess the size and patency of the portal or splenic veins, the size of the spleen, and the presence of ascites. Indeed, a fluid layer as shallow as 1 cm in the sitting position and a volume as small as 100 ml have been demonstrated by ultrasound and could be a spur to the aspiration of ascitic fluid.

Biliary Tract Disease

Gallstones

In the routine detection of gallbladder stones, ultrasound so far has no advantage over oral cholecystography, but its relative simplicity, the lack of radiation, and the fact that the patient need take no pills may well make it the first diagnostic step in the near future. Radiolucent and radiopaque stones can be detected with equal frequency, but the reported false negative rate for ultrasound of 10 percent, with a false positive rate of 1–5 percent[10-12] is greater than the false negative rate for oral cholecystography which runs about 3–5 percent, along with a much smaller false positive rate of about 1–2 percent. A more recent study by Crade et al[13] which relied on surgical and pathological assessment of gallbladder disease, found ultrasound to be even more accurate than oral cholecystography for the identification of gallstones if the classical findings of cholelithiasis were seen sonographically. The simplicity of ultrasound may shortly lead the clinician to forego any statistical advantages of the oral cholecystogram in favor of this noninvasive approach, reserving oral cholecystography for those patients in whom his clinical suspicions were not confirmed by standard X-ray. For the moment, however, ultrasound finds its place as the second diagnostic step—to confirm the possibility of gallstones in patients with faint gallbladder visualization on the standard single dose oral cholecystogram.

The distinctive appearance of gallstones at ultrasound is now well recognized, but the clinician still has many questions about the significance of "sludge" or echoes which move within the gallbladder without definitive evidence of stones; about the "false positive" echoes which have been reported; or how to deal with the patient whose gallbladder fails to visualize on double dose cholecystography, but who has a normal ultrasonogram. Finally, most of the time he does not need to know how well the gallbladder contracts or empties after a fatty meal except when deciding whether to use chenodeoxycholic acid to dissolve gallstones.

In some patients, ultrasound is already the standard first diagnostic approach to the gallbladder: 1) patients with predictable blocks to the absorption and excretion of oral cholecystographic dye, including patients with jaundice, hepatocellular disease, malabsorptive disorders, or motility disturbances of stomach or esophagus; 2) pregnant women with abdominal pain; 3) patients with acute cholecystitis or acute pancreatitis; 4) the rare patient with allergy to oral cholecystographic dye; 5) in patients with acute cholecystitis or pancreatitis, ultrasound is particularly useful to exclude gallstones.

Obstructive jaundice—dilated biliary ducts

By showing a dilated biliary tree, ultrasound now provides one of the first and most valuable clues in the jaundiced patient to distinguish intrahepatic from extrahepatic cholestasis. The overall accuracy of ultrasound in jaundiced patients, now reported at over 95 percent,[14] to some extent depends upon the kinds of patients studied. Ducts permanently obstructed from cancer of the bile ducts or pancreas, are apparently somewhat easier to detect than ones intermittently blocked by benign processes such as common duct stones. In the pioneer studies of Taylor and Rosenfield[14] as well as in other studies, errors were largely in patients with gallstones who were deemed to have intrahepatic cholestasis because of normal appearing ducts but who later proved to have stones causing obstruction. Still, Taylor and Rosenfield[14] found ultrasound to be diagnostic in 60 percent of patients with extrahepatic obstruction and contributory in another 30 percent. In another study of patients with obstructive jaundice,[15] a true positive rate of 100 percent and a false negative rate of 7 percent were extremely helpful, except that the false negatives were again all attributable to stone disease with intermittent duct obstruction. The appearance of normal ducts in such patients is usually attributed to a "fluctuating obstructive" process, and this factor may reduce the diagnostic potential of ultrasonography in this group of patients.

In the jaundiced patient, the clinician needs to diagnose treatable benign obstruction as early as possible. In patients with clinically apparent cancer, ultrasound may be "diagnostic" when looked at as the single diagnostic approach, but for the clinician who has already made that diagnosis, ultrasound ends up as "supportive" rather than diagnostic. The relatively small number of patients with stone disease so far reported and the absence of patients with common duct stones in many series leads us to await a final assessment of the place of ultrasound in the detection of common duct stones. If the absence of dilated ducts on ultrasound does not preclude "intermittent biliary tract obstruction", then the clinician may still need the more definitive help of percutaneous transhepatic cholangiography. So far, the exact level of obstruction still needs to be outlined by transhepatic cholangiography even when ductal dilatation is found by sonography. How quickly ducts dilate or how long they stay dilated after passage of a stone through the common duct are also matters for evaluation.

Published data and our own experience now make us turn to ultrasound as the first study for the jaundiced patient whose blood studies suggest cholestasis rather than hepatitis. The categorical presence of dilated ducts is the most help in reassuring the physician that he must go further. When dilated ducts are seen on ultrasound, percutaneous cholangiography is usually performed to delineate the site of obstruction clearly. If a pancreatic mass has been seen on ultrasound or if elevated amylase or lipase levels point to an obstruction of the ampulla or of the pancreatic duct itself, then endoscopic pancreatography can scrutinize the ampulla and duodenum and opacify the pancreatic duct. In the patient in whom dilated ducts are not seen, we currently assume the presence of intrahepatic cholestasis unless such clinical features as pain, chills, or fever suggest cholangitis. Liver biopsy usually is then carried out to prove the presence of a specific cause of intrahepatic cholestasis. Some clinicians prefer to observe the patient without biopsy for a period, particularly if a drug-induced or viral etiology is strongly suspected. In the patient without dilated ducts at ultrasound, in whom liver biopsy suggests extrahepatic cholestasis, either repeat ultrasound or transhepatic cholangiography is in order.

Cystic Lesions in the Abdomen

To tell whether an abdominal lesion is solid or cystic is not always easy on physical examination, and the ability of ultrasound to help in this distinction provides one of its more valuable assets. Radionuclide scans show solid masses or cysts as regions of decreased uptake; angiography usually clarifies the cystic nature of such a mass, but at the cost of some discomfort and time. Ultrasound is clearly the method of clinical choice, for the characteristic reflective cyst wall with its echo-free center is easily apparent even to the gastroenterologist and makes the differentiation of a cyst from a solid mass in the abdomen impressively useful especially, as we have pointed out, in the distinction of a pancreatic pseudocyst from a phlegmon. The following patient demonstrated the utility of sonography in the diagnosis of a cyst in a mass lesion thought to be solid in nature.

> A 58 year-old female nurse, an insulin-dependent diabetic of four years duration, and a nonalcoholic, came in with abdominal pain nausea and vomiting and was found on upper gastrointestinal examination to have a pyloric channel ulcer with outlet obstruction. An oral cholecystogram did not visualize, but the patient responded to conservative therapy, and a repeat X-ray examination suggested resolution of the aforementioned abnormalities. Three months after her first bout of abdominal pain, she was noted to have an alkaline phosphatase one and one half times normal, but felt well. Four months after her initial presentation, she experienced recurrence of her abdominal discomfort which was not associated with fever, chills or icterus. Over a four month period of time she had lost 15 pounds. On physical examination, a temperature of 100°, moderate hepatomegaly, and a right upper quadrant mass adjacent to, but separable from, the liver were noted. On physical examination this seemed to represent a solid lesion—either metastatic disease to the liver or an abscess of pancreatic or biliary etiology. An abdominal film suggested an abnormal air collection in the right upper quadrant (Figure 2a), and an abdominal ultrasound scan (Figure 2b) suggested a cystic lesion involving the liver, and a normal pancreas. At operation, a large abscess cavity involving the liver and containing several gallstones was found immediately behind a necrotic gallbladder.

The incidental demonstration of an asymptomatic cyst of liver or pancreas, or even kidney, may have little clinical value especially when there are no functional abnormalities. The clinician should not be stimulated by such a report to a flurry of clinical activity because an asymptomatic cystic lesion is almost never a carcinoma. Although the complications of nonparasitic cystic lesions of the liver include pain, infection, and obstructive jaundice, only rarely will their detection prove a boon to physician or patient in the absence

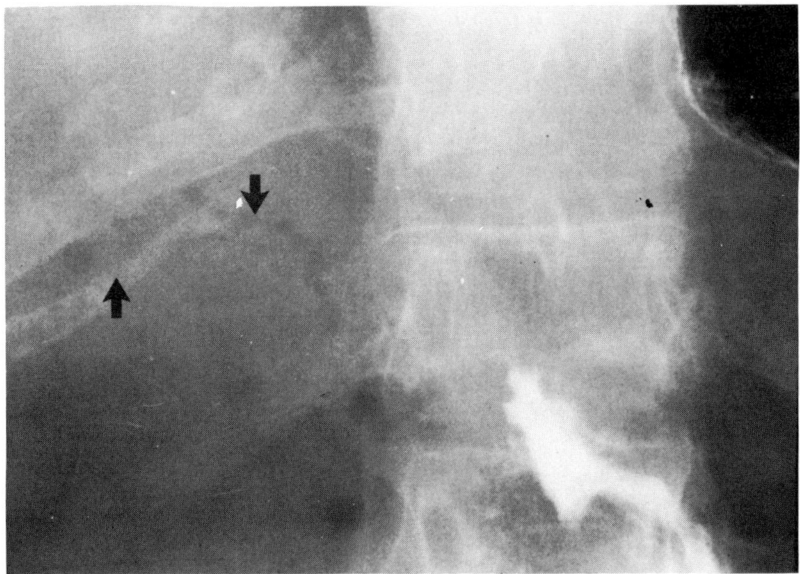

FIGURE 2. (a) Initial abdominal film demonstrating abnormal air collection in the right upper quadrant (black arrows).

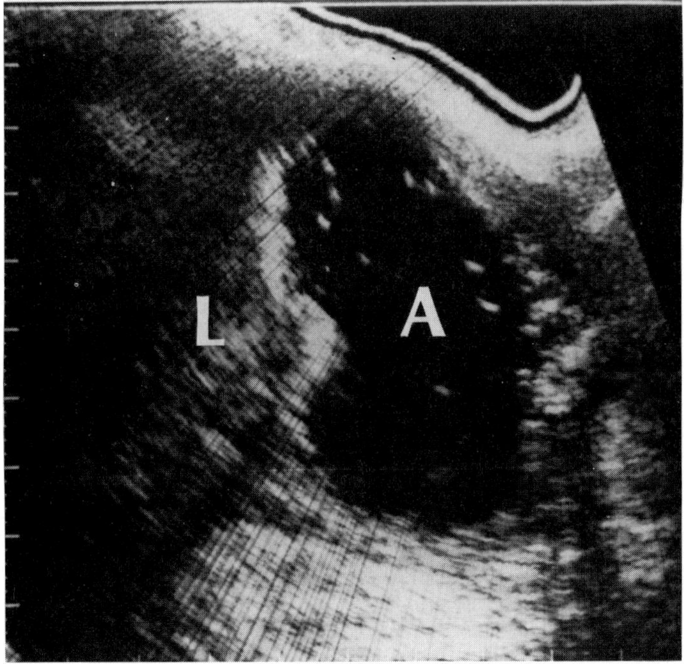

(b) Ultrasound demonstrating cystic lesion adjacent to liver. (L = liver; A = abcess.)

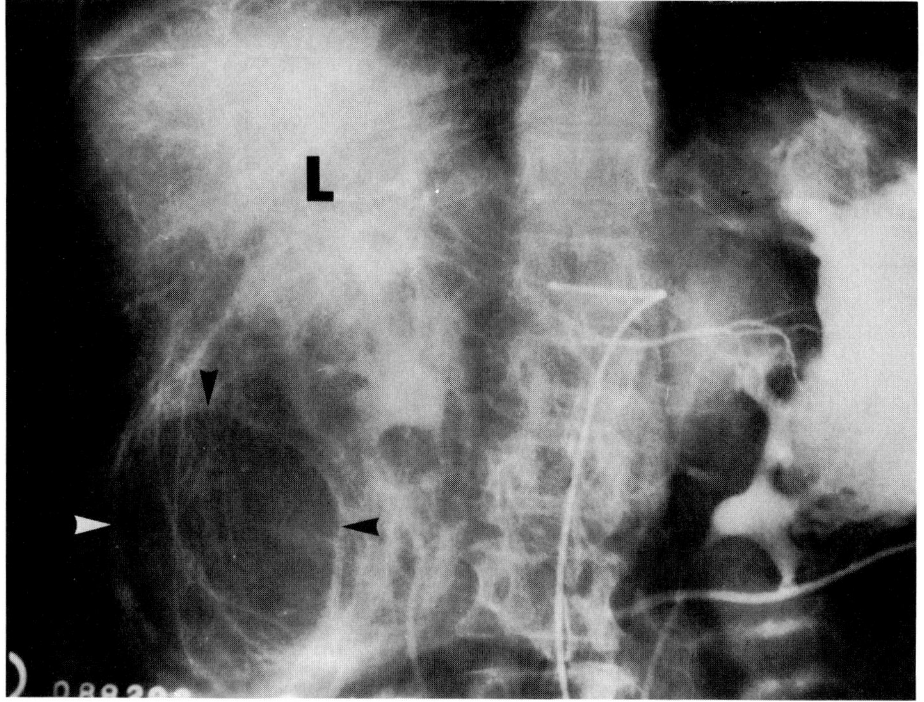

FIGURE 2 *continued.*

(c) Angiogram demonstrating cystic area (surrounded by arrows) involving liver (L).

of specific complaints. The same is true for the incidental renal cyst discovered by ultrasound which might lead to percutaneous aspiration with no advantage to the patient to compensate for the unpleasantness of the diagnostic studies.

Intra-Abdominal Abscess

Fever, abdominal pain, leukocytosis and abdominal signs often lead to the suspicion of an abdominal abscess. In the postoperative patient, however, and in the patient with Crohn's disease, detection of an intra-abdominal abscess may prove much more difficult. Localized mesenteric nodes or thickening of the bowel wall may simulate an abscess and corticosteroid therapy may mask the typical findings. Taylor et al[16] have reported correct identification of 36 of 40 subsequently proven abdominal abscesses (90 percent), so that we have come to rely on ultrasound for help in resolving this difficult clinical problem. However, some abscesses may be missed on ultrasound and the differentiation from hematoma or other fluid-filled compartment of the abdomen may prove difficult. Gallium scanning and labeled white cell scanning appear to be as sensitive as ultrasound in the detection of intra-abdominal abscesses, but are less specific. Much more clinical experience is needed for final assessment of how small an abscess can be identified and how often ultrasound is really helpful. At present we rely on ultrasound as a guide but do not regard it as categorical.

Intra-Abdominal Vascular Disease

Ultrasound can be helpful in the detection of an aortic aneurysm which may mimic other intra-abdominal masses, and can reassure the clinician that a pulsatile abdominal mass is not an aneurysm. More important, it has taught the clinician how inaccurate the physical examination can be and that aneurysmal calcification is present on plain abdominal X-ray in only 42 percent of patients with abdominal aneurysm.[17] Ultrasound now seems preferable to angiography in the screening of a patient with an aortic aneurysm.

To Resolve Clinical Ambiguity

Ultrasound helps resolve ambiguity in the patient with cancer. Palpation of the liver may confirm a clinical impression of metastases, but cannot give histologic details. What remains to be shown is whether ultrasound provides anything more than "very sensitive fingers", that is, whether it can distinguish one mass lesion from another sufficiently well to make histologic confirmation unnecessary. Radionuclide imaging is regarded as nonspecific because defects on liver scans may represent cysts, abscesses, metastases, avascular areas, or regenerative nodules in the cirrhotic patient. Unless ultrasound yields more precise information, it will not replace liver biopsy in the patient without a known tumor in the liver. While present studies suggest that this may be true, we currently find its best use in the follow-up of the hepatic masses in patients with known cancer and increasingly it is replacing radionuclide imaging.

Problems of detection remain, however. For example, Smith et al[19] correctly identified liver abnormalities in 14 of 15 patients (93 percent) who developed metastases from carcinoma of the breast, but there was histologic confirmation in only 9 of these. Ultrasound was superior to radionuclide scanning, which correctly identified 78 percent of patients with known metastases, with a false positive rate of 23 percent. This contrasts with ultrasound's false positive rate of only 5 percent. A study in patients with Hodgkin's disease[20] in whom the findings were confirmed at operation are more disappointing to the clinician looking to avoid liver biopsy. Radionuclide imaging gave a correct positive rate of 50 percent and a correct negative rate of about 80 percent. Ultrasound was slightly more accurate, but not enough for absolute clinical reliability. Taylor and Carpenter[21] found ultrasound to be diagnostically contributory in 92 percent of 120 patients with carcinoma, while radionuclide scanning was helpful in only 48 percent. More impressive, however, was their low combined false negative and false positive rate of 8 percent for ultrasound, contrasting with 27 percent for nuclear scans. Sullivan et al[22] aptly demonstrated the accuracy of ultrasound in helping to clarify equivocal radionuclide scans of the liver, demonstrating similar degrees of sensitivity for each, but much higher specificity for ultrasound (74 percent vs 93 percent).

The clinician must assess the clinical utility of ultrasound in patients who do *not* have overt metastases. For example, we need to know how often patients will have a new diagnosis of metastases made by ultrasound, and how that determination contributes to patient care; whether, for example, ultrasound is more sensitive than a rise in alkaline phosphatase or even quantitation of the carcinoembryonic antigen levels.

Ultrasound appears to be particularly useful in patients with an equivocal radionuclide scan, not only in resolving ambiguity about hepatic defects but in giving more definitive information; yet we need to determine how useful such information will be. It seems likely that an important role of ultrasound will be to identify patients without metastases who do not need liver biopsy, to follow the course of metastases, or to detect their development during therapy. Further experience is needed to confirm the notion that ultrasound detects metastases in the liver with over 90 percent accuracy. Specifically we need to know how early and how reliably this can be done.

As A Screening Study

Ultrasonography is used in two different ways as a screening study, particularly where there is a suspicion of cancer:

a) In the patient with such nonspecific symptoms as weight loss or longstanding abdominal pain or even cancer phobia or depression, the clinician too often orders an ultrasound study "to be sure", or simply as a diagnostic placebo to reassure the patient. This has been the case with every new diagnostic technique over the past years, from carcinoembryonic antigen to angiography and panendoscopy. The remarkable sensitivity and precision of ultrasound, however, leads to even greater problems, for the discovery of cysts or other lesions which are not expected generates many more morphological studies than the clinical circumstances would demand. The following case demonstrates how sonography used to examine one portion of the abdomen can uncover unexpected findings in another.

> A 51 year old restaurant owner with a 20 year history of esophageal reflux was seen because of increasing symptoms associated with a 20 pound weight loss, and depression. He was a teetotaler, and showed nothing abnormal on physical examination. A panendoscopic examination showed esophagitis. The patient was treated with a strict antireflux regime, but continued to experience pain, and lost an additional 15 pounds. An ultrasound examination was carried out at that time, primarily to screen for a pancreatic neoplasm. It demonstrated a normal

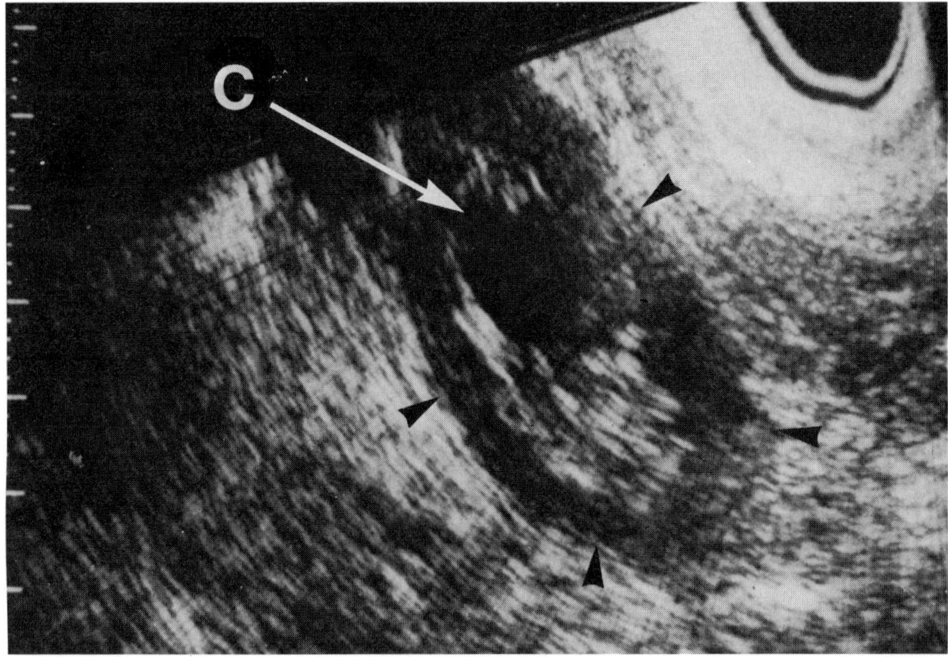

FIGURE 3. (a) Ultrasound scan showing cystic area (c) in hilum of left kidney (bordered by arrows).

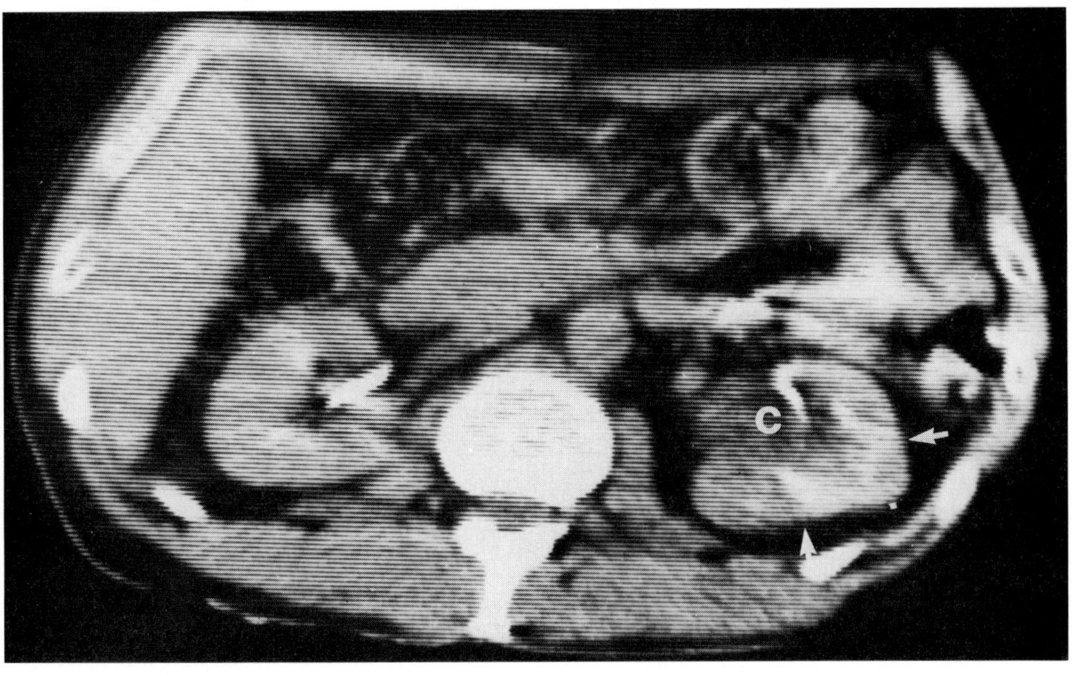

(b) CT scan showing cystic area (c) in hilum of left kidney (bordered by arrows).

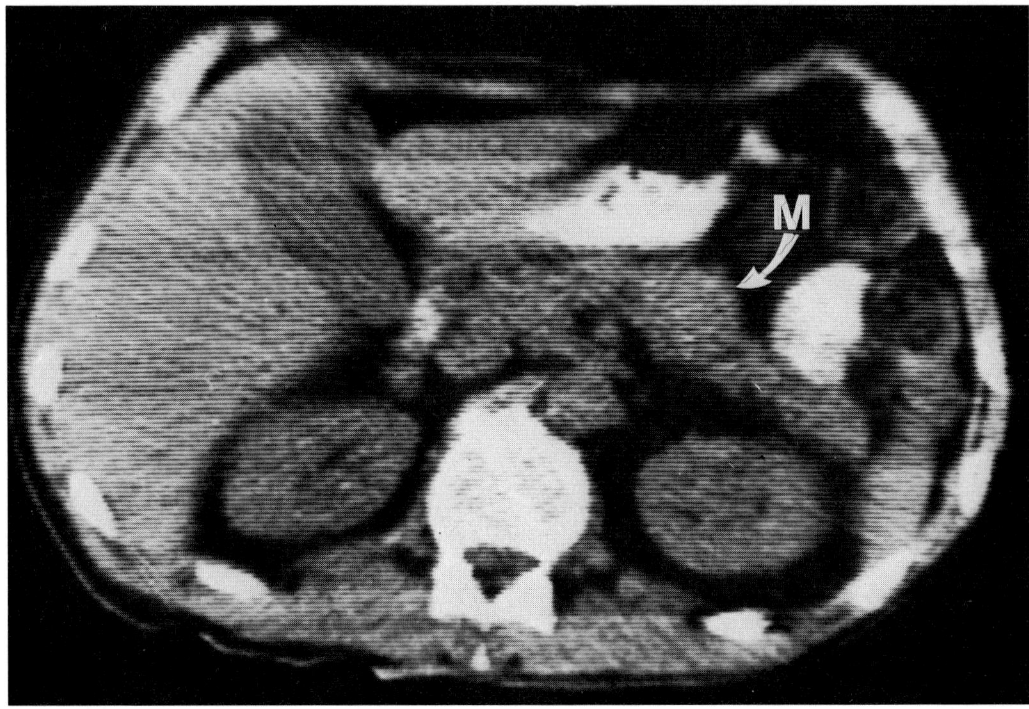

FIGURE 3 *continued.*
(c) CT scan with possible pancreatic mass (M).

pancreas, but a cystic area appeared in the calyceal area of the left kidney (Figure 3a). A CT scan was performed to confirm the cystic area in the left kidney (Figure 3b) and demonstrated such, but was also thought to demonstrate a lesion in the tail of the pancreas (Figure 3c). To help resolve the question of a pancreatic mass, abdominal angiography along with endoscopic retrograde pancreatography were performed, both of which suggested normality of the pancreas.

b) More appropriately helpful is the use of ultrasound as a screening test in the patient with specific abdominal pain suggestive of pancreatic cancer or other lesion. In such circumstances, ultrasound can guide the clinician to a more aggressive and more important diagnostic approach, though a normal ultrasound view of the pancreas or other organs in the abdomen can not yet serve as the "perfect" screening test to guarantee absence of disease. Until such time, we suspect that the lazy clinician who turns to ultrasound simply as a way of getting rid of the talkative patient or reassuring the worried healthy patient or who simply uses ultrasound as a screening test without talking to his patients, will uncover lesions which are not always clinically significant and whose discovery will occasion increased financial and diagnostic outlay. By such comments we do not suggest that the careful clinician should not use ultrasound as a screening modality, but we do wish to emphasize the danger.

Generally, the results of most screening studies will depend upon the kinds of patients chosen, as we have emphasized throughout this review. The following case suggests how ultrasound can be helpful when applied to the appropriate patient as a screening test.

> A 75 year-old retired businessman had had a four month history of lower abdominal pain. After a normal sigmoidoscopy, upper gastrointestinal series and barium enema, he was treated symptomatically, but gradually became depressed and lost 30 pounds. Physical examination and routine laboratory data were normal. The main clinical problem appeared to be depression, but an abdominal ultrasound was ordered, and raised the question of a lesion in the tail of the pancreas (Figure 4a). Subsequently, a CT scan (Figure 4b) and ERCP (Figure 4c) were performed, both suggesting carcinoma of the tail of the pancreas. The diagnosis was confirmed at the time of surgery.

The clinical gastroenterologist will look at ultrasound *specificity* and *sensitivity* in the light of how it shortens or simplifies his diagnostic approach,

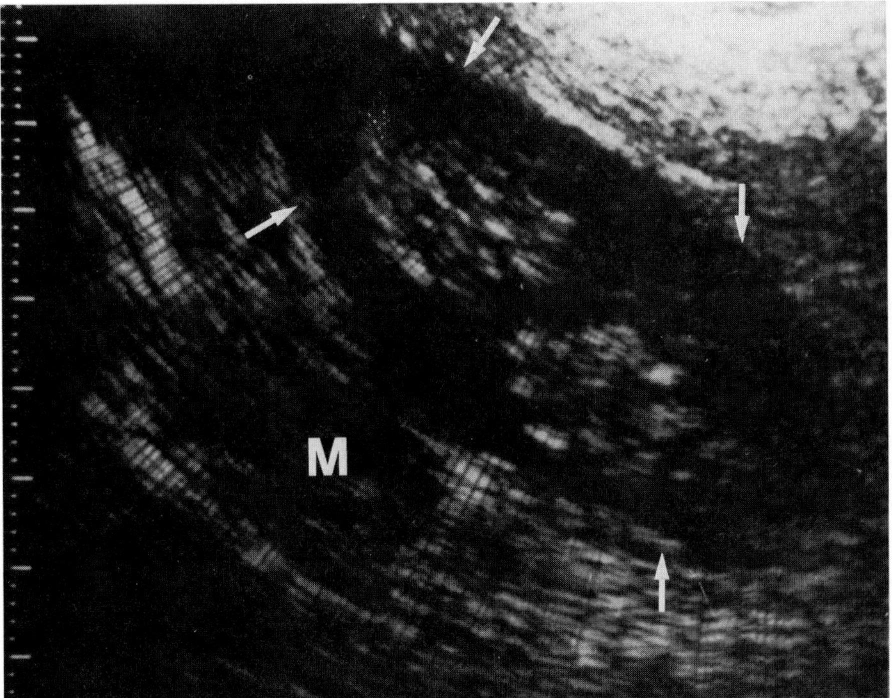

FIGURE 4. (a) Ultrasound scan suggesting mass lesion in the pancreatic tail (M). The outline of the left kidney is arrowed.

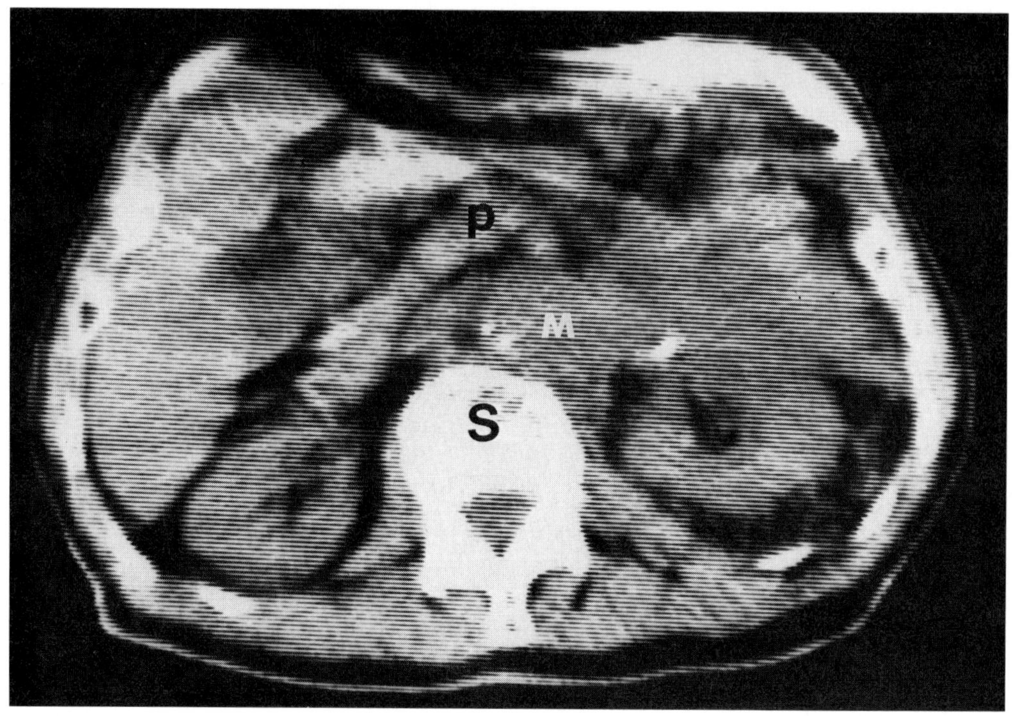

FIGURE 4 *continued.*

(b) CT scan demonstrating mass lesion (M) and pancreatic displacement (p). (S = spine.)

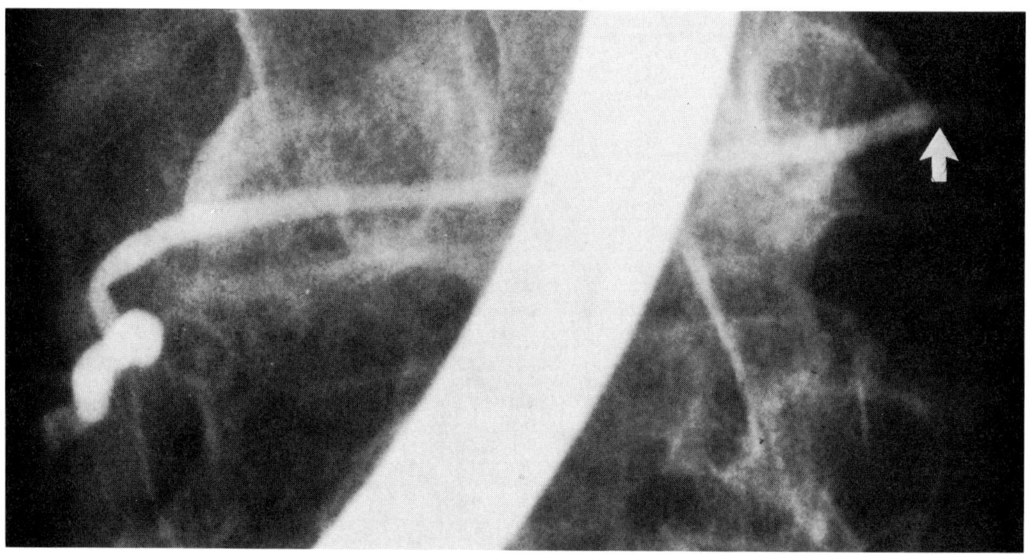

(c) Endoscopic retrograde pancreatography demonstrating cut-off of distal pancreatic duct (point of arrow).

what further burdens it places upon the patient, and how he would have acted without it. Very often, nevertheless, ultrasound offers a relatively inexpensive noninvasive technique and especially in the middle-aged or older person with complaints of organic portent, the physician is fully justified in using ultrasound to look for occult lesions in the liver, biliary tract, pancreas, or retroperitoneal areas.

The Follow-Up Of Previously Identified Lesions

Ultrasonography is now frequently used to monitor the status of a number of quantitatable lesions. The first patient presented in this text is an example of how the ultrasound can be used in regards to a pancreatic pseudocyst, and its use in following cystic lesions, including most abscesses, in the abdominal cavity. The difficult monitoring of an abdominal aortic aneurysm's size can be done accurately with ultrasound. Some patients with cancer are being followed by ultrasound to assess their response to therapy. Whether ultrasonography will be able to separate the surrounding inflammation necrosis and desmoplasia from tumor, or be as efficacious with all tumor types when used in assessment of response to therapy remains to be seen. The types of pathology that can be followed by ultrasonography will primarily be limited by the ability of this modality to accurately and reproducibly measure a given abnormality.

Miscellaneous

There are now a number of other clinical settings in which sonography has been utilized more as an exhibition of diagnostic agility than for any clinical utility. This includes the detection of such cystic lesions as duplication cyst, or such mass lesions as hypertrophic pyloric stenosis, gastric cancer or hematomas involving intraabdominal organs. Much of the time these are simply demonstrations of the sophistication of the ultrasonographer rather than examples for serious clinical use. Whether ultrasound will challenge the pappilotomist in his ability to extract gallstones or the chemotherapist now busily dissolving them with chenic acid remains to be seen, but fragmentation of a gallstone by ultrasound has already been reported!

Summary

Ultrasound has proven to be a welcome aid to the clinician, and because of its relatively cheap, safe,[23] rapid, and noninvasive approach, it has quickly earned a firm place in the diagnostic armamentarium. The clinician would like to know about observer variation, variations in one machine or technician to another, and especially how much reliability at one institution can be transferred to another. At Yale we have been fortunate in our extraordinarily reliable and intuitive echography, but so far there are not enough skilled echographers for confidence to be universal. As gastroenterologists, however, we consider ultrasound a boon in the detection of cystic lesions in the abdomen, dilated hepatic ducts, and in the detection of gallstones. Many further areas remain for exploration.

ACKNOWLEDGEMENTS:
We would like to thank Drs Kenneth Taylor and Arthur Rosenfield for sonograms, Dr. Robert Lowman for radiographs, and Sue DeSantis and Carolyn Kocher for preparation of the manuscript.

References

1. DiMagno EP, Malagelada JR, Taylor WR, Go VLW: A prospective comparison of the current diagnostic tests for pancreatic cancer. N Engl J Med 297:737–742, 1977.
2. Levitt RG, Geisse GG, Sagel SS, Stanley RJ, Evens RG, Koehler RE, Jost RG: Complementary use of ultrasound and computed tomography in studies of the pancreas and kidney. Radiology 126:149–152, 1978.
3. Husband JE, Meire HB, Kreel L.: Comparison of ultrasound and computer-assisted tomography in pancreatic diagnosis. Br J Radiol 50:855–862, 1977.
4. McCormack LR, Seat SS, Strum WB: Pancreatic carcinoma: survival following detection by ultrasonic scanning. JAMA 238:240, 1977.
5. Hancke S, Holm HH, Koch F: Ultrasonically guided percutaneous fine needle biopsy of the pancreas. Surg Gynecol Obstet 140:361–364, 1975.
6. Smith EH, Bartrum RJ, Chang YC, Dorst J, Lokich J, Abbuzzese A, Dantono J: Percutaneous aspiration biopsy of the pancreas under ultrasonic guidance. N Engl J Med 292:825–828, 1975.
7. Doust BD, Pearce JD: Gray scale ultrasonic properties of the normal and inflamed pancreas. Radiology 120:653–657, 1976.
8. Kressel HY, Margulis AR, Gooding GW, Filly RA, Moss AA, Korobkin M: CT scanning and ultrasound in the evaluation of pancreatic pseudocysts: a preliminary comparison. Radiology 126:153–157, 1978.
9. Goldberg BB, Goodman GA, Clearfield HR: Evaluation of ascites by ultrasound. Radiology 96:15–22, 1970.
10. Arnon S, Rosenquist CJ: Gray scale cholecystosonography: an evaluation of accuracy. Am J Roentgenol 127:817–818, 1976.
11. Bartrum RJ, Crow HC, Foote SR: Ultrasonic and radiographic cholecystography. N Engl J Med 296:538–541, 1977.
12. Prian GW, Norton LW, Eule J, Eiseman B: Clinical indications and accuracy of gray scale ultrasonography in the patient with suspected biliary tract disease. Am J Surg 134: 705–711, 1977.
13. Crade M, Taylor KJW, Rosenfield AT, de Graaff CS, Minihan P: Surgical and pathological correlation of cholecystosonography and cholecystography: accuracy in 145 patients. Am J Roentgenol 131:227–230, 1978.

14. Taylor KJW, Rosenfield AT: Gray scale ultrasonography in the differential diagnosis of jaundice. Arch Surg 112:820–825, 1977.
15. Conrad MR, Landay MJ, Janes JO: Sonographic 'parallel channel' sign of biliary tree enlargement in mild to moderate obstructive jaundice. J Roentgenol 130:279–286, 1978.
16. Taylor KJW, McI Wasson JF, de Graaff CS, Rosenfield AT, Andriole VT: Accuracy of gray-scale ultrasound diagnosis of abdominal and pelvic abcesses in 220 patients. Lancet 1:83–84, 1978.
17. McGregor JC, Pollock JG, Anton HC: The value of ultrasonography in the diagnosis of abdominal aortic aneurysm. Scot Med J 20:133–137, 1975.
18. Gilby ED, Taylor KJW: Ultrasound monitoring of hepatic metastasis during chemotherapy. Br Med J 1:371–373, 1975.
19. Smith IE, Taylor KJW, McCready VR, Powles TJ, Bondy PK: A comparison of gray-scale ultrasound with other methods for the detection of liver metastasis from breast carcinoma. Clin Oncol 2:47–53, 1976.
20. Glees JP, Taylor KJW, Gazet JC, Peckham MJ, McCready VR: Accuracy of gray-scale ultrasonography of liver and spleen in Hodgkin's disease and the other lymphomas compared with isotope scans. Clin Radiol 28:233–238, 1977.
21. Taylor KJW, Carpenter DA: Comparison of ultrasound and radioisotope examination in the diagnosis of hepatobiliary disease. In Ultrasound in Medicine, eds. White DN, Brown RE, New York, Plenum Press, 2:159–167, 1974.
22. Sullivan DC, Taylor KJW, Gottschalk A: The use of ultrasound to enhance the diagnostic utility of the equivocal liver scintigraph. Radiology 128:727–732, 1978.
23. Baker ML, Dalrymple GV: Biological effects of diagnostic ultrasound: a review. Radiology 126:479–483, 1978.

Ultrasound Evaluation of Diffuse Liver Disease

JASON C. BIRNHOLZ

We will assume that "diffuse liver disease" implies a process which is extensive and anatomically poorly defined, without sharp delineation between histologically normal and abnormal parenchyma. Focal lesions such as cysts, abscesses, vascular malformations and primary and secondary neoplasms (with the possible exception of diffuse hepatoma) are excluded by this definition, but are discussed in Chapter 3 of this issue. A simple etiological classification of diffuse liver disease which pertains to ultrasonic differential diagnosis is:

1. parenchymal dysfunction secondary to vascular disorders
   a. right-sided congestive heart failure
   b. hepatic vein thrombosis
   c. portal vein thrombosis, pylephlebitis
2. hepatitis
   a. acute: viral, toxic (i.e. alcoholic, drug-related)
   b. chronic
3. parenchymal infiltration
   a. fatty liver
   b. granulomatous diseases
   c. amyloid
   d. leukemia, lymphoma, myeloid metaplasia
   e. lipid/glycogen storage diseases
4. cirrhosis
5. parenchymal dysfunction secondary to biliary tract disease
   a. obstruction
   b. cholangitis

Functional disorders of hepatic metabolism, such as the Gilbert or Crigler-Najjar syndromes and disorders particular to pediatric populations will not be considered herein, and discussion of biliary tract disorders is presented separately (see Chapter 7).

Examination Technique

The examination includes subjective estimate of hepatic and splenic volume (or other indicator of overall organ size), observation of the shape of the liver, and assessment of hepatic tenderness. Diagnostically useful vascular structures which are visualized are the first and second order hepatic and portal veins, and the splenic vein. The pleural and peritoneal spaces are inspected for effusion and, finally, there is detailed imaging of portions of the hepatic and splenic parenchyma. Since diffuse processes are not confined anatomically, parenchymal assessment need not require thorough sampling of the entire hepatic volume. A portion of the right lobe is always accessible ultrasonically via intercostal portals at mid- and anterior axillary line levels, and transverse views through these portals with the subject supine are recommended. An oblique intercostal view medial to the anterior axillary line, oriented along the course of the portal vein, is optimal for surveying the porta hepatis. Occasionally, the porta hepatis is visualized most readily in an oblique subcostal plane with the subject in a left decubitus position. Proximal hepatic veins are visualized either with midline transverse views angulated cephalad or with a left decubitus sagittal section. A lateral intercostal scanning portal is also satisfactory for assessment of splenic parenchyma, although, since the spleen is relatively posterior in position, it is often necessary to turn the subject onto his right side for probe placement.

Electronic sector scanning (phased array) imaging is well suited to the hepatic evaluation because the small probe size permits intercostal viewing. The anatomic structures already mentioned are located and optimal scanning planes are determined expeditiously. In addition, the mechanical properties of the liver may be inferred from observation of shape changes (or shape invariance) during respiration or palpation, as seen on high speed (real-time) imaging. Conventional static imaging has an advantage, at present, in viewing the parenchymal architecture, because of flexibility in transducer choice. Transducer selection will be discussed later. In addition, digital scan conversion systems provide some measure of operator control of certain facets of signal processing.

Parenchymal Texture

Ultrasound imaging is a means of mapping tissue elasticity gradients. For the most part, this corresponds to portraying the concentration, structural configuration and physiological state of collagen. The collagen—reticular skeleton of the liver provides an abundance of acoustic scattering centers, which appear as a textured background in the final image. Each visceral organ has a characteristic texture pattern (Figures 1 and 2). Visual recognition of normal

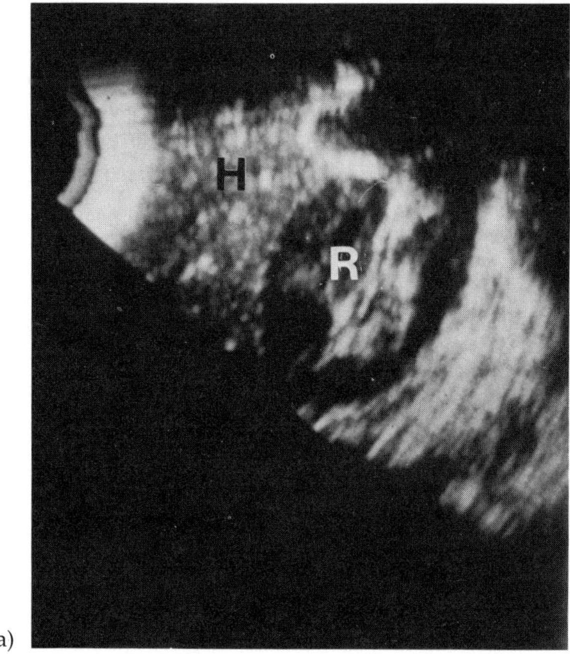

(a)

FIGURE 1. (a) Comparison views of hepatic (H) and renal (R) architecture. (b) Hepatic (H) and splenic (S) textures. Subject in Figure 1a has lymphoma without hepatic infiltration.

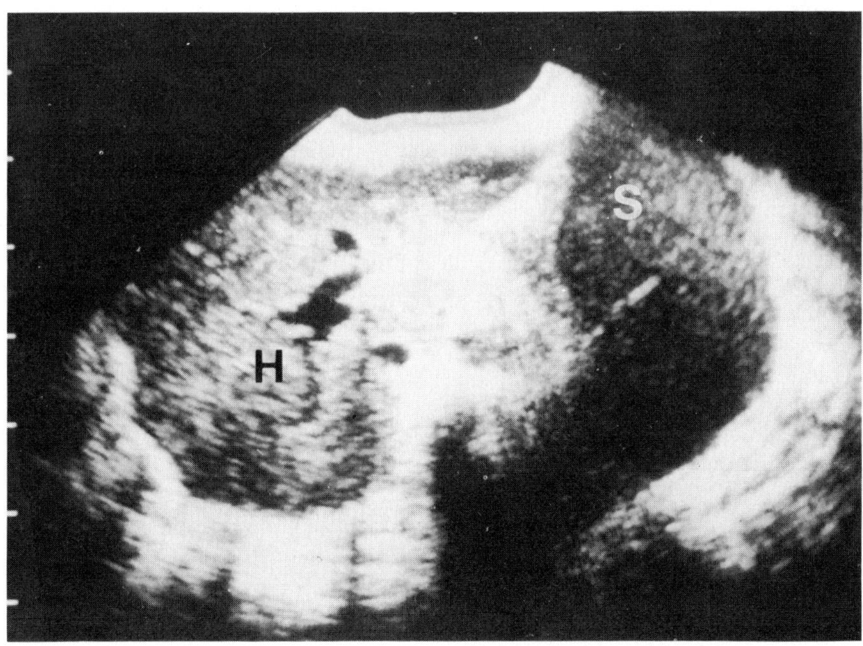

(b)

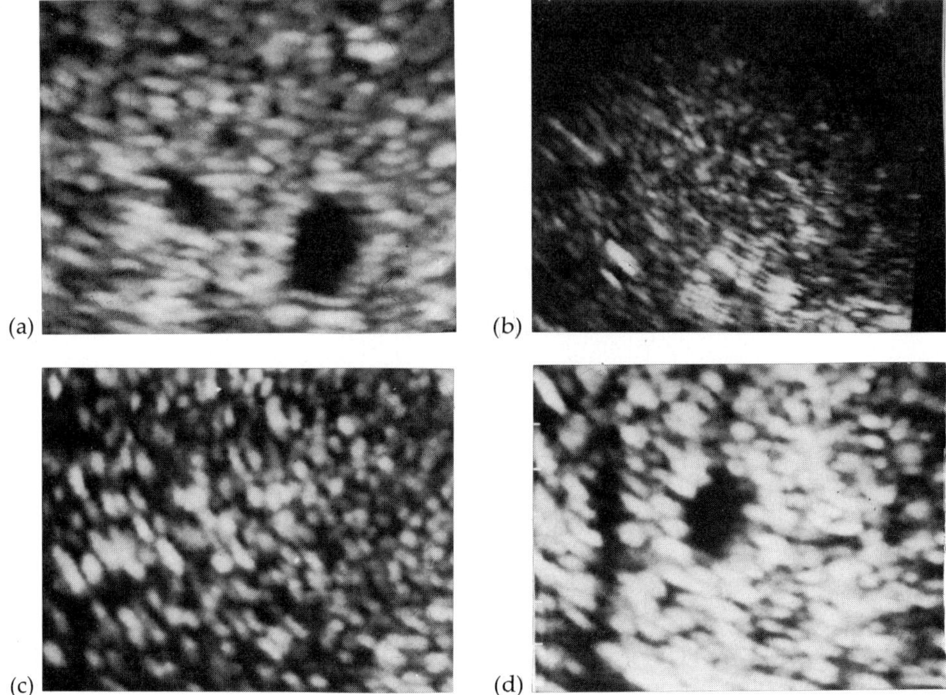

FIGURE 2. Hepatic texture patterns at the focal region of a 2.25 MHz transducer, magnified 8 times. Pattern (a) is normal; (b) is fatty degeneration; (c) is combined fatty changes and fibrosis; and (d) is predominant fibrosis.

and pathologic texture patterns is central to the ultrasonic diagnosis of diffuse liver disease.

Ultrasonic parenchymal texture represents the histologic macrostructure of the region, modified by certain aspects of the acoustic pulse—tissue interaction and a variety of instrument performance factors. Different "textures" can be produced by scanning the same target region with different commercial systems or with variant use of one instrument. The physical foundations which underlie parenchymal texture appearance must be considered before individual experience in one facility can be standardized or generalized in clinical usage.

The term "texture" applies (visually and photographically) to small-scale luminance variations in a background region. Inclusive technical definition and characterization of texture patterns is difficult, although there has been progress in determining the statistical features of textures for computer-based pattern recognition procedures. Descriptive qualities which are useful in practical ultrasound usage are the average sizes of the echo targets, which vary from *fine* to *coarse*, and the population density, which varies from *sparse* to *dense*. Textures may be *random* or *patterned*, and they may be *uniform* (regular) or *non-uniform* (heterogeneous) for population density distribution and/or luminance (signal amplitude or gray scale).

Gray scale display features vary according to the size, shape, and configuration of individual parenchymal targets as well as on the specific relationship between the dimensions of those structures and the spectral characteristics of the interrogating pulse. The texture display for closely packed populations of those targets also varies according to the number of those structures which combine to form a single "reflector" in the final image, i.e., the volume of tissue insonified in each range compartment. The spatial and spectral features of the beam are, therefore, integral considerations in texture portrayal; consequently, transducer selection cannot be haphazard. As center frequency is increased, all other factors being unchanged, attenuation increases; however, the absolute number of scattering structures which are detected increases disproportionately, the backscatter profiles of previously detected targets are altered, and the overall dynamic range (i.e., gray-scale contrast) decreases. These observations underscore the fact that it is difficult to compare textures obtained with transducers which differ in size, focusing and spectral characteristics (same manufacturing line); which differ in construction (different manufacturers); or which are excited differently (different instrument lines). Within any individual facility, comparable views should be obtained with the same transducer for each case in which texture discrimination is desired.

The spectrum of the pulse changes with depth during tissue propagation. Tissues act as "low pass" acoustic filters, which is in some ways equivalent to "hardening" of an X-ray beam as it traverses a tissue path. Since texture rendition is related to pulse spectrum, it is anticipated that there may be a gradation of texture with depth. It is appropriate, therefore, to study comparable depth regions when evaluating parenchymal textures in different subjects or when forming a library of texture patterns based on practical experience. It is probable that multiple reverberation artifacts contribute to the apparent texture pattern as well. These will depend in some measure on intrinsic tissue macrostructure as well as the character of intervening tissue material. This suggests that body habitus may play a role in texture appearance and that library patterns should be subclassified by superficial extrahepatic tissue features as well as the depth and transducer factors already mentioned.

Research suggests that the connective tissue at the lobular level of organization is the principal tissue determinant of hepatic parenchymal texture.[1] The average dimension of this periodic structure is slightly more than 1 mm, or slightly more than the center wavelength of a 2.25 MHz pulse. Since the reflecting structure and pulse wavelength are of a similar order of magnitude, slight change in either (i.e., tissue pathology which compresses or expands the normal structure, or transducer change in the 1–4 MHz range), will have a particularly marked effect on the detection and display of parenchymal architecture. This suggests that any one transducer will not necessarily be optimal for studying both normal and abnormal livers.

The previous discussion has not included the potential effects of receiver and display section signal processing schemes. Receiver bandwidth and dynamic range are usually sufficiently broad for the transducer input signal. The maximum display dynamic range, however, is limited, so that the dynamic range of the input signal must be compressed in some fashion. The mode of signal compression (and other signal processing techniques which are incorporated in commercial imaging systems) is not standardized. Since these have a profound influence on the final image, it can be appreciated that texture comparison of images derived with systems having disparate signal processing methods may pose additional interpretive difficulties. The instrument considerations already mentioned have assumed ideal operational performance; in practice, however, texture display will be degraded when beam position sensing accuracy, incorrect velocity compensation, and display device focus or dynamic range are suboptimal. These factors are relevant to the scanning strategy which is used, namely simple versus compound, peak detection versus integration. Simple scanning, peak detection operation is most satisfactory for the majority of units in service.

The eye and brain must also be included in the image chain when considering the factors influencing texture portrayal. There is considerable evidence that there are significant perceptional disparities between the white-on-black and black-on-white display modes for texture identification.[2, 3] White-on-black is superior in this regard. In addition, in order to achieve reproducibility in evaluating textures in different subjects, consistency must be maintained in display screen brightness and contrast, display size, photographic technique, and the background illumination of the photograph or display screen during interpretation. It is often helpful to subselect a texture region at a specific depth (in the region of the transducer focus) and magnify that zone such that no anatomical details are obvious. Texture alone may then be evaluated.

These many factors indicate that, at the present time, each clinical facility should develop a fixed operational scheme and its own library of normal and pathologic texture patterns. Individual examples will be presented in this review as a guide rather than as a general reference.

Diffuse Liver Disease With Normal Parenchymal Architecture

Quite profound levels of jaundice may be seen with acute right-sided congestive heart failure. Hepatomegaly is the typical presenting feature of congestive failure in childhood, and it should not be forgotten that jaundice and hepatomegaly may dominate the clinical presentation of congestive failure in the adult. This situation should be considered when there is sudden onset of painless jaundice without prodromal or other historical features suggestive of viral or toxic hepatitis. The liver is large and tender. The parenchymal architecture is "normal" throughout and the inferior vena cava (IVC) and intrahepatic veins are distended. Respiratory variations in the caliber of the IVC and hepatic veins are abolished. The spleen is usually normal in size and architecture. Ascites and pleural effusions are typical.

Hepatic volume and functional compromise correlate with hepatic venous pressure. Substantial and very rapid reduction in hepatic size is observed when venous pressure can be reduced promptly. This is perhaps most evident in the younger subject with normal cardiac function, in whom right-sided failure is due to pericardial disease. In the older subject, intrinsic cardiac disease may limit the speed with which improvement is accomplished and a component of low output from coincident left-sided heart failure will contribute to hepatic decompensation (via hypoxic centrizonal necrosis). Repeated and prolonged episodes of congestive failure may also initiate permanent damage leading to cardiac cirrhosis. Hepatic vein pressure is notably high with tricuspid insufficiency, in which case pulsations of the hepatic veins are a regular finding. Pulsations of the liver itself are found when regurgitant flow is great. This condition is documented ultrasonically by observing the flow pattern of microbubbles induced by the forceful manual (or automatic pressure) intravenous injection of a bolus of saline. Clearance of the bubbles from the right atrium is slow, regurgitant flow from the right ventricle into the right atrium may be seen, and microbubbles are ejected into the hepatic veins.

The use of electronic sector scanning methods for real-time examination have shown that hepatic veins are always visualized in the normal subject. When there is massive ascites, the veins may not be seen (even after deep inspiration), probably because of some component of extrinsic hepatic compression. In the absence of massive ascites, inability to visualize the hepatic veins, therefore, suggests the possibility of hepatic vein thrombosis, i.e., the Budd-Chiari syndrome. Conversely, this possibility warrants particular consideration when a subject with any condition which facilitates coagulation sustains sudden hepatic functional decompensation. When repeated ultrasound attempts do not disclose the hepatic veins, the simplest procedure for confirmation or exclusion of hepatic venous occlusion is plain radiography of the right upper quadrant, after intravenous CO_2 injection, with the subject in the left decubitus, Trendelenberg position.

The appearance of the liver with granulomatous infiltration may be normal. The texture pattern is usually normal with viral hepatitis, although hepatosplenomegaly occurs, and the liver is notably tender. With some viral strains (e.g., Coxsackie) and with chronic active hepatitis, pleural and/or pericardial effusions are common.

Alcoholic Liver Disease

Parenchymal liver disease related to alcoholism accounts for the largest category of cases referred for examination. Fatty change and cirrhosis will be considered as distinct groups, although various combinations of the two processes are typical.

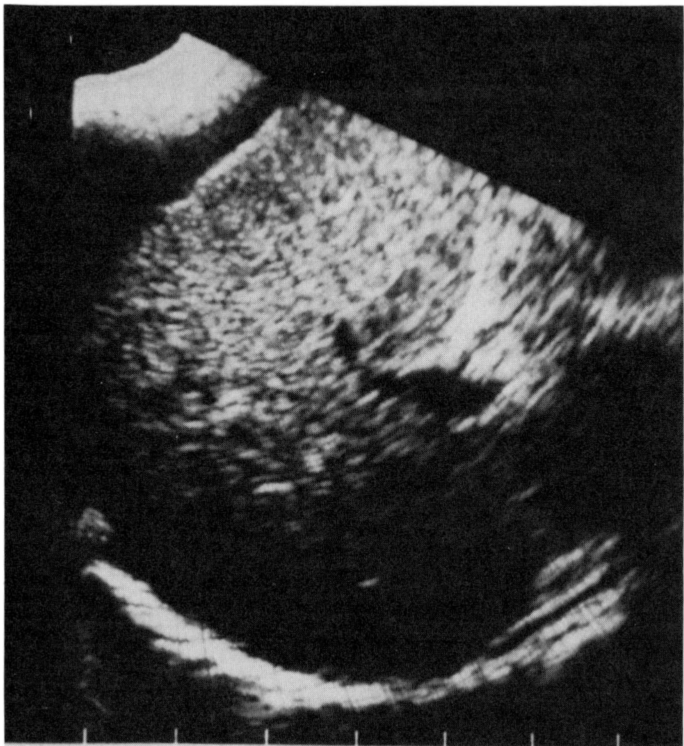

FIGURE 3. Attenuation with depth is pronounced when there is significant fibrosis. This subject has micronodular cirrhosis with acute hepatic decompensation following spree drinking.

Fatty change may or may not progress to cirrhosis. Fat deposits are diffuse and vary from 4 to 10 μ, occasionally coalescing into 100 μ diameter fatty "cysts", which are still below separate resolution limits. In the early stages of acute fatty degeneration, the liver is large, smooth and pliable. Attenuation is normal to decreased. The texture pattern is a fine mesh of delicate and individually separated echoes. There is slight to moderate amplitude heterogeneity, with the subjective impression that there is a bi- or trimodal amplitude distribution.

There are several pathologic lesions which have an identical final common result in cirrhosis. Necrosis and hepatic cellular collapse and septal formation with fibroblast and vascular proliferation are the relevant features with the ultrasonic concomitant of increased population density of parenchymal echoes and increased attenuation (due to increased scatter) (Figure 3). With typical Laennec's cirrhosis, the hepatocyte population is reduced to numerous small nodular islands separated by thick, fibrous septi, i.e., the hobnail pattern. In addition to becoming more closely spaced, individual echoes are

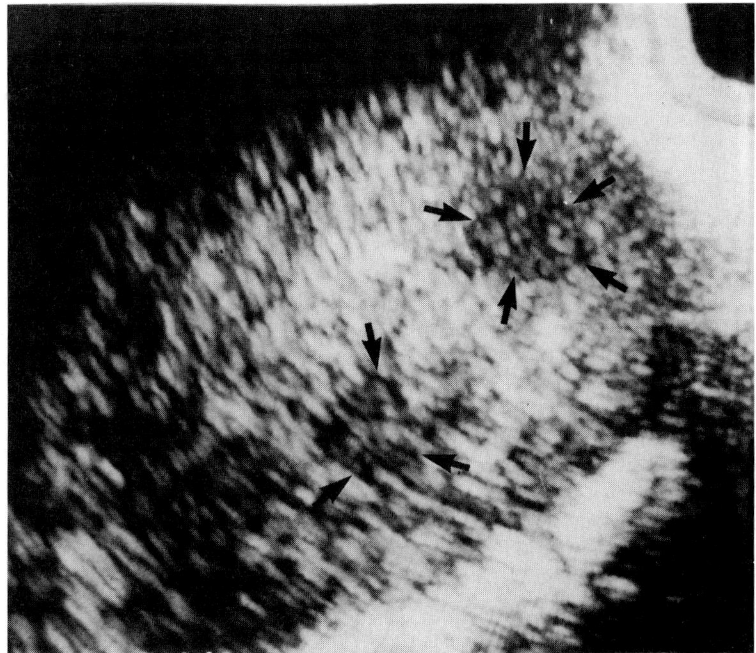

FIGURE 4. Regenerating nodules (arrows) appear as ill-defined zones which are hypoechoic relative to the coarse, echodense background of significant fibrosis. The absence of sharp marginal distinction, desmoplastic reaction and central necrosis aid in distinguishing these nodules from focal metastatic lesions.

also coarser. The progression of cirrhosis is often patchy, so that zones of closely-spaced, high-amplitude echoes are often intermingled with more normal appearing parenchyma. This structural heterogeneity is the most characteristic diagnostic feature.

The end-stage cirrhotic liver is small and firm, and it does not exhibit shape changes with respiration or manual compression. Hepatic marginal irregularities are typical with macronodular cirrhosis. Regenerating nodules are hepatocyte islands with considerably less collagen content than surrounding affected liver (there is also absence of a central vein structure so that the collagen vascular substructure differs from that of normal liver). These regions may appear as hypoechoic islands within the hepatic parenchyma (Figure 4). They are less well marginated than focal neoplastic lesions.

Ascites is easily demonstrated ultrasonically. Some ancillary information may be gained by noting that a predominantly fatty liver will float in a transudate, while a fibrotic liver will sink dependently. Portal venous and splenic changes with portal hypertension may be deduced from extant angiographic works and will not be discussed in this chapter.

Diffuse Infiltrative Liver Diseases

The occurrence of diffuse metastatic lesions, all of which are less than 2 mm in diameter, is an unusual finding with small cell tumors such as melanoma and sarcoma. Most often with metastatic disease, at least a few discrete nodules will be identified, and these may clarify the diagnosis, providing the imaging system has sufficiently good resolution. In the rare diffuse case, the parenchymal texture may be expected to be quite coarse. Lymphoma may occur either as a diffuse small cell infiltration or as discrete nodules (most often with Hodgkin's disease). The appearance may be entirely normal in early stages of the former process.

With diffuse and extensive small cell infiltration, as with some of the leukemias, an occasional lymphoma, or (most often) myeloid metaplasia, the liver is large, attenuation is notably decreased, and the texture pattern is abnormal with uniform amplitude distribution.

Comment

Present, subjective experience indicates that the parenchymal texture pattern conveys anatomical and pathologic information which is highly specific. No information is available concerning the sensitivity of the method (i.e., the false-negative rate). A prospective analysis of this factor, within the many constraints of data acquisition already indicated, is necessary (and finally possible).

Computer methods of data analysis may be particularly helpful in grading hepatic parenchymal patterns. Mountford and Wells[4] and Taylor and Milan[5] have shown that simple time domain techniques derived from A-scan recordings can provide reliable measures of population density and average amplitude characteristics of parenchymal echoes; Fraser, Kino, and Birnholz[1] have shown that, with some additional signal processing methods, the periodicities and other statistical features of the echo distribution may also be extracted from the same data. These preliminary approaches to quantitative assessment of the parenchymal texture pattern are relevant to routine clinical usage, since they can be incorporated into the postprocessing functions of newer digital scan conversion imaging systems which are now available.

References

1. Fraser J, Kino GS, Birnholz JC: Cepstral signal processing in diagnostic ultrasound. In Linzer M, ed: Proceedings of the Second Conference on Ultrasonic Tissue Characterization, National Bureau of Standards, June 1977 (In press).

2. Bartlesan CJ, Breneman EJ: Brightness perception in complex fields. J Opt Soc Am 57: 953–957, 1967.
3. Mezrich JJ, Birnholz JC: Contrast reversal influence on structure perception (In preparation).
4. Mountford RA, Wells PNT: Ultrasonic liver scanning: The A-scan in the normal and cirrhosis. Phys Med Biol 17:261–269, 1972.
5. Taylor KJW, Milan J: Differential diagnosis of chronic splenomegaly by grey scale ultrasonography: clinical observations and digital A-scan analysis. Br J Radiol 49:519–525, 1976.

Demonstration of Focal Liver Disease by Ultrasound and Computed Tomography

HYLTON B. MEIRE
JANET HUSBAND

Both X-ray computed tomography (CT) and ultrasound produce an anatomical display of the liver, but since each technique uses a different form of energy (X-radiation and sound waves) they measure different physical properties. The images produced by the two systems are influenced by a variety of technical factors which affect the anatomical detail obtained.[1-3]

Technical Considerations

Since X-ray computed tomography and ultrasound are rapidly developing techniques, significant advances in equipment are likely during the next few years. At the present time, the capital outlay and running costs of CT scanners are approximately ten times those of ultrasound machines; but CT has the advantage of automation, whereas high-resolution ultrasound machines are at present manually operated. The results obtained with an ultrasound scanner are therefore highly dependent upon the skill of the operator. However, this does permit interactions between operator and equipment which optimize the display of the normal anatomy or abnormality in many cases. Both techniques require supervision by an experienced radiologist during the examination if optimal results are to be obtained.

Both systems produce a tomogram of the patient 3–13 mm in thickness. The image obtained with CT is in the transverse plane, whereas ultrasound can produce an image in almost any plane. With CT it is possible to produce a vertical reconstruction of an image but, at the moment, the poor resolution of these limits the clinical value of this facility. Improved resolution can be obtained by overlapping scans, but at the price of a much higher dose of ionizing radiation.

Data acquisition time is almost instantaneous with ultrasound, whereas with CT both the scan time and computer processing time result in a certain delay before an image is displayed. The scan time with new CT machines is now only a few seconds and the processing time with many of the scanners currently available is of the order of 1–2 minutes. Since the data acquisition time with ultrasound is extremely short, there is little movement of intrahepatic structures during a single sweep scan; in addition, each structure is sampled only once. This results in a high spatial resolution so that it is possible to recognise intrahepatic structures, such as hepatic veins, as small as 2 mm in diameter. With CT, spatial resolution to this degree is not possible at the present time because multiple sampling of the same cross section is made during each scan, and some movement of internal structures is inevitable. In terms of pathology, however, the spatial resolution of both systems is probably similar. With ultrasound, it is usually possible to detect metastases of about 2 cm in diameter,[4] although smaller lesions may occasionally be detected under ideal circumstances. We have correctly diagnosed metastases less than 1 cm in diameter in cases where more than three such lesions were present. With CT, the same order of spatial resolution is possible but the ability to detect a lesion is highly dependent on the degree that its density differs from that of normal liver. Tumors no greater than 1 cm in diameter have been displayed,[5] but in the majority of instances it is difficult to detect a metastasis smaller than 2 cm. The advent of faster scan times should improve spatial resolution,[6] but in order to obtain adequate information a higher dose of X-radiation is again required.

Computed tomography demonstrates the entire cross section of the abdomen at the level of the slice. The relationship of the liver to other organs and structures is clearly shown and associated or incidental pathology may be detected, including lesions in bone or lung. Ultrasound produces a limited view of the area of interest on each scan and very few other anatomical landmarks are included in some images.

The main limitation of ultrasound is the complete reflection of sound waves by gas and bone. Successful liver examinations are possible in over 90 percent of patients, but problems do arise when the liver is situated high under the costal margin or if there is excessive bowel gas. It is virtually impossible to display 100 percent of the liver by ultrasound scanning, the lateral extremities usually being the most difficult areas to visualize. Obesity also causes difficulty, particularly in obtaining adequate images of the posterior aspect of the right lobe.

Liver CT scans are similarly degraded by various artifacts.[5, 7] Streak artifacts are produced by the ribs in a significant number of patients; by metal clips; by high density contrast medium; and by gas in moving bowel. Cardiac pulsation is a frequent cause of artifacts near the dome of the diaphragm. Respiratory movement degrades the CT image,[8] but can be eliminated by performing all scans during arrested respiration in those machines where a scan time of 20 seconds or less is available.

Both CT and ultrasound are affected by the partial volume effect, which can result in the inability to detect a lesion or in its misinterpretation. If a lesion occupies the whole thickness of the slice, then the reconstructed image represents the attenuation of X-rays, or reflection of sound waves, of that structure alone. However, if the lesion only partially occupies the slice, then the recorded image represents a composite of normal tissue and the lesion. The attenuation of the X-ray beam and the reflected sound waves thus represent a contribution from normal tissue as well as from the lesion, and it is possible to mistake a cyst for a solid tumor, or to interpret the scan as normal.[5] Computed tomography has the disadvantage of using X-radiation. The dose of X-radiation varies according to the equipment used and field size. Using the EMI Whole Body Scanner (CT 5005) with a 13-inch field size, the total absorbed skin dose for an examination of ten slices is approximately 3.5 rads.

Instrumentation

Our experience has been obtained using commercial gray-scale ultrasound machines (Nuclear Enterprises Diasonograph) and EMI Whole Body Scanners.

Examination Technique

Ultrasound

Liver ultrasound examination is generally performed with the patient lying supine. The anterior abdominal wall is coated with a suitable contact medium—we use olive oil—and scans are performed manually whilst holding the transducer in contact with the skin.

In general it is necessary to perform scans during suspended inspiration to bring the liver down below the costal margin. Inspiration may be dispensed with in patients with low diaphragms or hepatomegaly. A series of longitudinal scans are performed across the area of the liver and spaced about 1 cm apart. Wider spacing will reduce one's chances of detecting small focal defects. A single sweep of the transducer is preferred[9] since this prevents degradation of resolution owing to movement of the liver during the cardiac cycle. We also employ a series of transverse scans to assist in visualization of the lateral extremities of the liver, the whole examination normally taking about ten minutes.

We do not prepare the patient for examination since we have found no regime which significantly reduces bowel gas.[10]. If a suitable drug or regime is discovered it would be used only prior to a repeat scan on patients with a failed initial examination.

Good gray-scale display is essential for all liver ultrasound examinations and the transducer frequency selected should be the maximum consistent with penetration to the back of the right lobe. This will usually be 3.5 MHz for thin or average patients and 2.25 MHz for the larger patients.

Careful attention is necessary to equipment output, sensitivity and swept gain controls to ensure that an even distribution of medium gray echoes is obtained throughout the liver depth. The precise means of achieving this varies with different types of equipment and will not be discussed here, but failure to obtain correct adjustment of the equipment will result in an increase in both false positive and false negative examinations. This is a major disadvantage of current ultrasound equipment. Conversely, the major advantage of ultrasound is that it can be repeated as often as necessary with no known hazard to the patient or operator.

A variety of automatic real-time ultrasound scanners is becoming available, and several have now achieved both the gray scale and resolution necessary to examine the liver adequately. These will certainly have a role to play in the future of liver ultrasonography.

CT Scanning

The EMI Whole Body Scanner (CT 5005) has a scan time of 20 seconds; the slice thickness is 13 mm and the image is displayed on a 320 × 320 matrix. Prior to the examination, a conventional radiograph of the chest and abdomen is taken, using a slit beam of X-rays to avoid geometrical distortion.[11] A metal marker is placed on the suprasternal notch so that the position of the slices can be related to the anatomical vertebral level. Prior to the examination an anticholinergic agent is given to reduce peristalsis and eliminate streak artifacts as much as possible. We currently give Buscopan (Hyoscine-N-butyl bromatum) 20 mg intramuscularly five to ten minutes before the procedure.

Slices are taken through the liver at 1.5 cm intervals from the dome of the diaphragm to the tip of the right lobe, during suspended respiration. A total of 10 to 12 slices is usually required, which takes approximately 30 to 40 minutes to complete.

Intravenous, urographic contrast agents may be used to increase the attenuation value of normal liver tissue. They may, therefore, be used to increase the contrast between normal liver and a suspected lesion, thus making identification easier.[12]

This is certainly true with avascular tumors and cysts, but those tumors with a high vascular component may also take up contrast. In this situation, the lesion becomes more difficult to detect.[5] The window settings on the viewing console also influence contrast between different densities; narrowing the window width decreases the gray scale between different densities and increases the contrast. It is clearly important to interrogate the scan data at various window settings since lesions not clearly visible with a wide window may be obvious using a narrow window setting. This simple maneuver

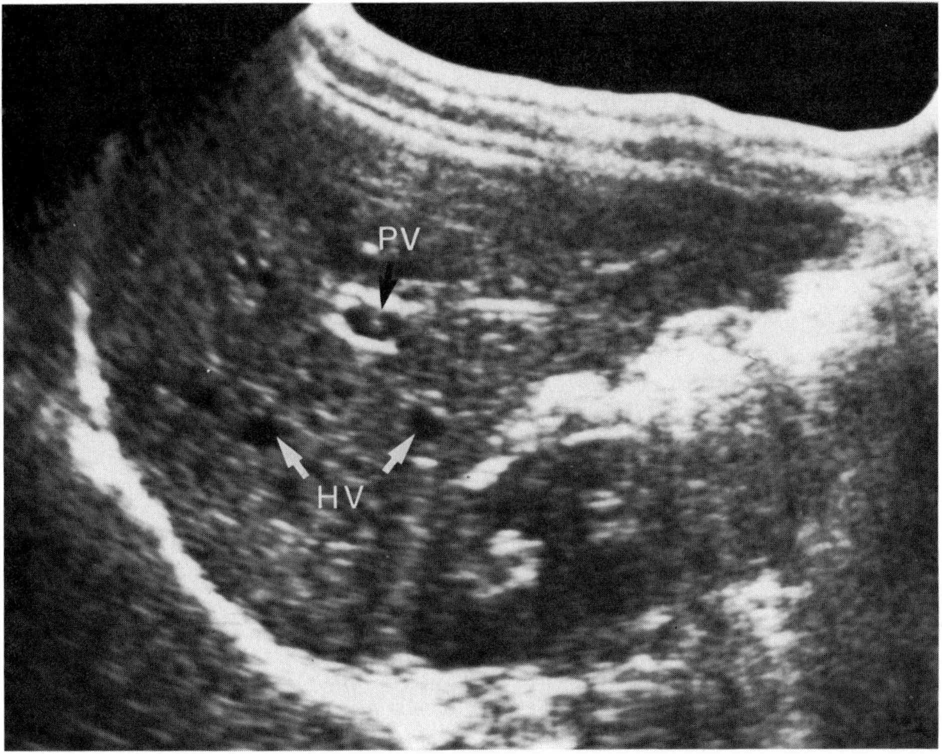

FIGURE 1. Longitudinal scan of normal right lobe of liver. The portal vein branches (PV), have echogenic walls, in contrast to the hepatic veins (HV).

frequently precludes the use of intravenous contrast which is not only unpleasant for the patient, but prolongs the total examination time.

Normal Anatomy

Ultrasound

The liver parenchyma produces a medium gray homogeneous echo pattern. Intrahepatic portal vein radicles and hepatic veins are seen more clearly than on the CT scan (Figures 1 and 2). The portal veins are differentiated from hepatic veins by the high-level echoes reflected from their walls. Hepatic veins, on the other hand, appear as echo-free rings or tubular structures with no surrounding high-level echoes,[13] and their communication with the inferior vena cava can easily be established by choice of a suitable scanning plane (Figure 2). This is very much easier and more rapid with real-time scanners. As with CT, it is possible to identify the individual liver lobes and ligaments. Rarely, the caudate lobe shows an echo pattern different from that produced by the remainder of the normal liver parenchyma. With both systems it is cur-

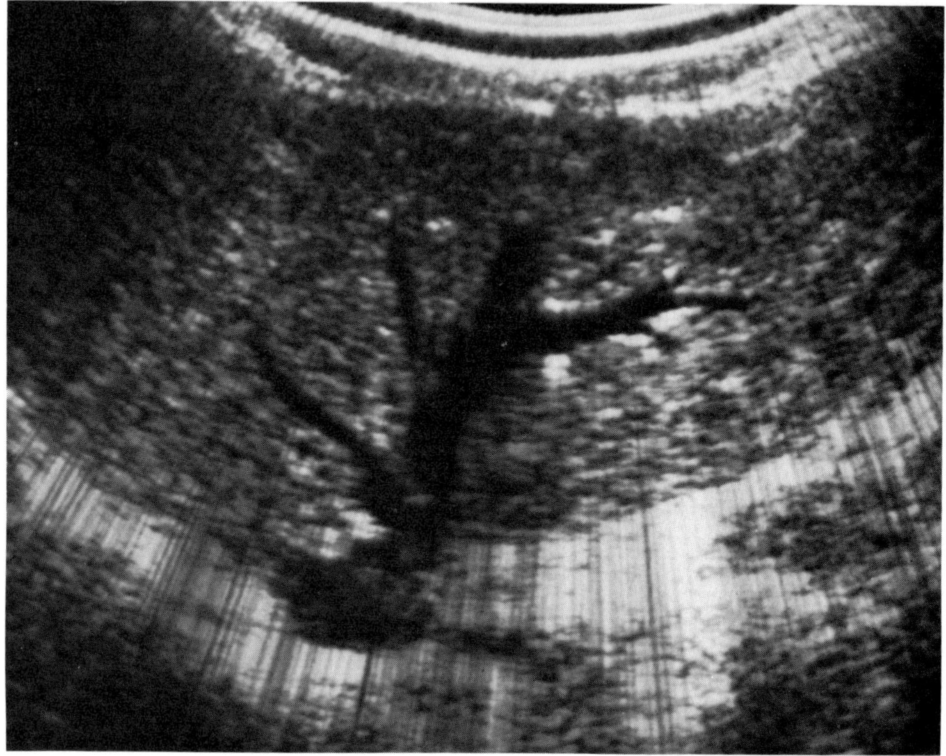

FIGURE 2. Transverse scan of liver. The scanning frame has been angled until the hepatic venous system is optimally displayed.

rently impossible to identify normal-sized intrahepatic bile ducts; however, they are clearly displayed by both techniques if dilated, and with CT if they contain air. Since air completely reflects sound waves, it is not possible to outline air-containing ducts with ultrasound; but they do produce a characteristic echo pattern, and may interfere with sound penetration sufficiently to cause difficulty in displaying the posterior portion of the liver.

The hepatic artery and common bile duct are now quite often seen in patients who are not obese or unduly gassy.[14]

The gallbladder is equally well shown by both ultrasound and CT. There is little difficulty in distinguishing this structure from a space-occupying lesion.

Computed Tomography

The normal liver parenchyma has a relatively homogeneous appearance, with a density higher than that of other intra-abdominal organs (e.g., kidney, pancreas, small bowel).[15] The CT number varies from approximately 20 to 40

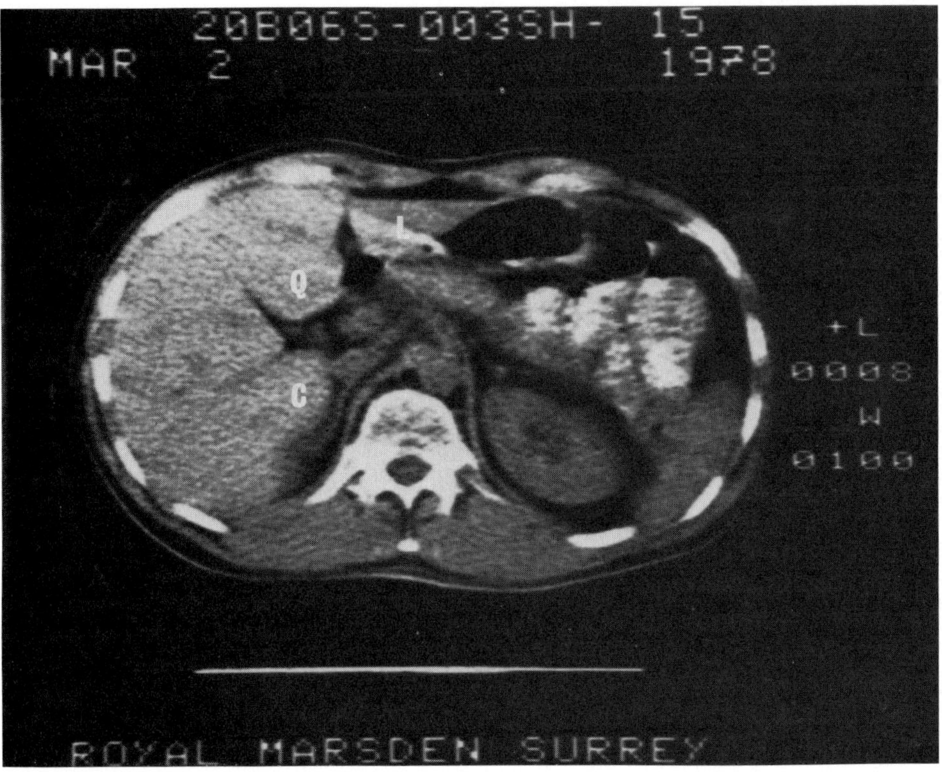

FIGURE 3. Normal liver. Left lobe (L); quadrate lobe (Q); caudate lobe (C).

(EMI units). Since the entire cross section of the liver is shown on each slice, it is possible to identify the individual lobes clearly (Figure 3). There is considerable variation in size and shape of the normal liver; occasionally a Riedel's lobe, extending to the pelvic brim, may be recognised. The shape of the left lobe is more variable than that of the right; it may be triangular, flattened or more rounded. The right lobe, occupying the major part of the right side of the abdomen, is more constant in position and shape. Anteriorly, the fissure for the falciform ligament and ligamentum teres can be identified because it has a low density. Similarly, the fissure containing the gastro-hepatic ligament and ligamentum venosum can be identified posteriorly. The caudate lobe produces a bulge on the medial aspect of the right lobe between the inferior vena cava and the fissure for the ligamentum venosum. The quadrate lobe is also frequently seen on the CT scan lying anterior to the liver hilum and caudate lobe. In patients with sufficient intra-abdominal fat, it is possible to identify the common bile duct and hepatic artery within the porta hepatis.

The major vascular channels are seen as areas of decreased density in those patients in whom the CT attenuation values for blood are significantly lower

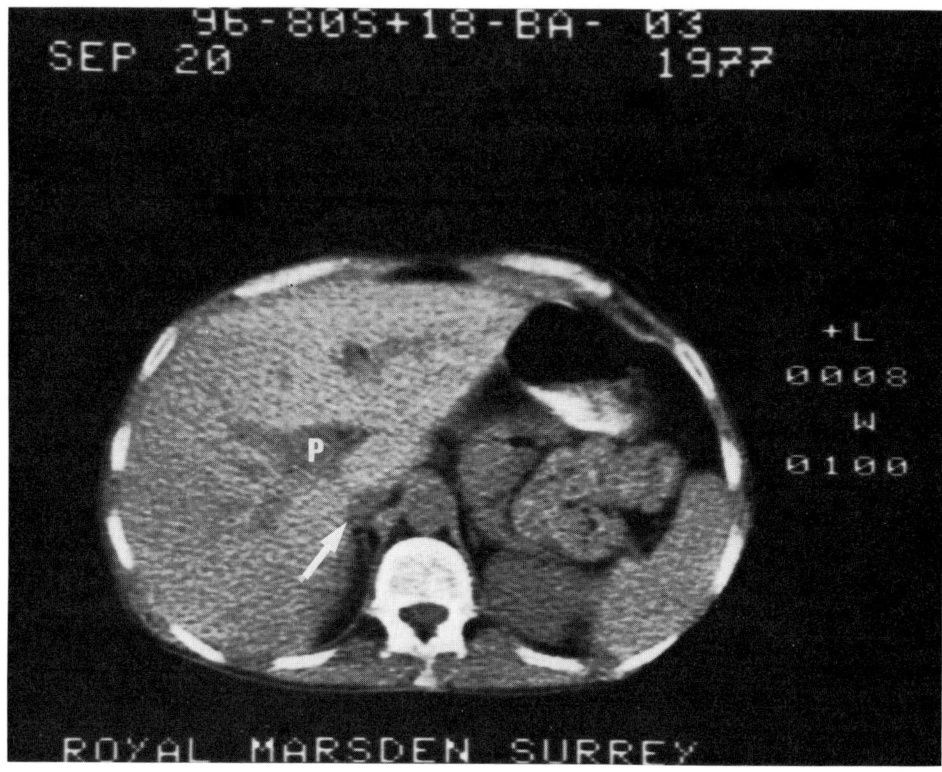

FIGURE 4. Normal liver. The major vessels appear as areas of low density. Portal vein (P); inferior vena cava (arrow).

than those for normal liver (Figure 4). However, if the CT value for blood falls within the range of the normal liver, vessels are not identified.[16, 17]

The major portal veins appear as low-density circular or tubular structures which are more obvious near the porta hepatis than peripherally. On serial slices, these structures can be shown to converge towards the hilum. The inferior vena cava can also usually be identified in the posterior aspect of the right lobe. Using the Varian Six Second Body Scanner, Harell et al,[6] reported that the liver contains many small oval, or Y-shaped areas of lower density than normal liver parenchyma in two-thirds of normal patients. They conclude that these structures are probably portal vein branches, hepatic veins or other parts of the portal triad. Normal-sized intrahepatic bile ducts are not seen on the CT scan.[18]

Focal Liver Disease

The major role of both ultrasound and computed tomography of the liver probably lies in the evaluation of the space-occupying lesion and obstructive jaundice. In this comparative review we are solely concerned with the capabilities and limitations of these techniques in relation to space-occupying lesions. The exact place of each system in terms of clinical management, and their relationship to each other in terms of diagnostic accuracy still requires further evaluation. In our experience of one hundred patients who have had both ultrasound and CT examinations of the liver, the diagnostic accuracy is similar. There was agreement between the ultrasound and CT findings in 85 percent of patients. In 7 percent the ultrasound examination was unsuccessful owing to overlying bowel gas, and in 2 percent the CT scans were undiagnostic owing to streak artifacts. In the remaining 6 percent an incorrect diagnosis was made either by ultrasound or CT. However, in this group the correct diagnosis was made in each patient by one of the techniques.

Both ultrasound and computed tomography are not only able to detect many space-occupying lesions, but also usually provide information regarding their composition.[19, 20] It is therefore possible to identify tumors, both benign and malignant, primary and secondary, and to distinguish these from cysts and abscesses in many instances. Levitt et al,[12] have assessed the diagnostic accuracy of CT in the liver and biliary tract in a group of 226 patients. Space-occupying lesions were detected in 46 patients with proved liver lesions. The nature of the space-occupying lesion was correctly diagnosed in 78 percent. Earlier studies in smaller groups of patients[8, 17] have also indicated that CT is accurate in the diagnosis of space-occupying lesions. Errors occur when the attenuation values of a lesion do not vary significantly from surrounding normal liver, or when partial volume averaging affects the true attenuation reading. This is a particular problem when the lesion is smaller than 2 cm in diameter. If the attenuation value of a focal lesion falls in the range intermediate between that of a cyst (0 to 10 Hounsfield units) and a tumor (10 to 15 Hounsfield units below that of normal liver) then the true composition of the lesion may be impossible to diagnose with CT. Another source of error is the presence of artifacts which may render detection of an abnormality impossible.

Ultrasound is also accurate in the diagnosis of space-occupying lesions of the liver.[21] With this technique, a variety of different appearances may be seen in both primary and secondary tumors. There is also a loose correlation between ultrasound appearances and tumor type.[22, 23] With computed tomography, however, the vast majority of liver tumors have a lower CT attenuation value than normal liver.[24] The only exceptions are tumors containing calcium, such as primary hepatomas or metastases from an osteogenic sarcoma, colloid carcinoma of the colon or ovarian tumors.

Malignant Tumors

Primary malignant hepatomas are extremely rare in the United Kingdom and our experience is therefore limited. The tumor usually produces localized or

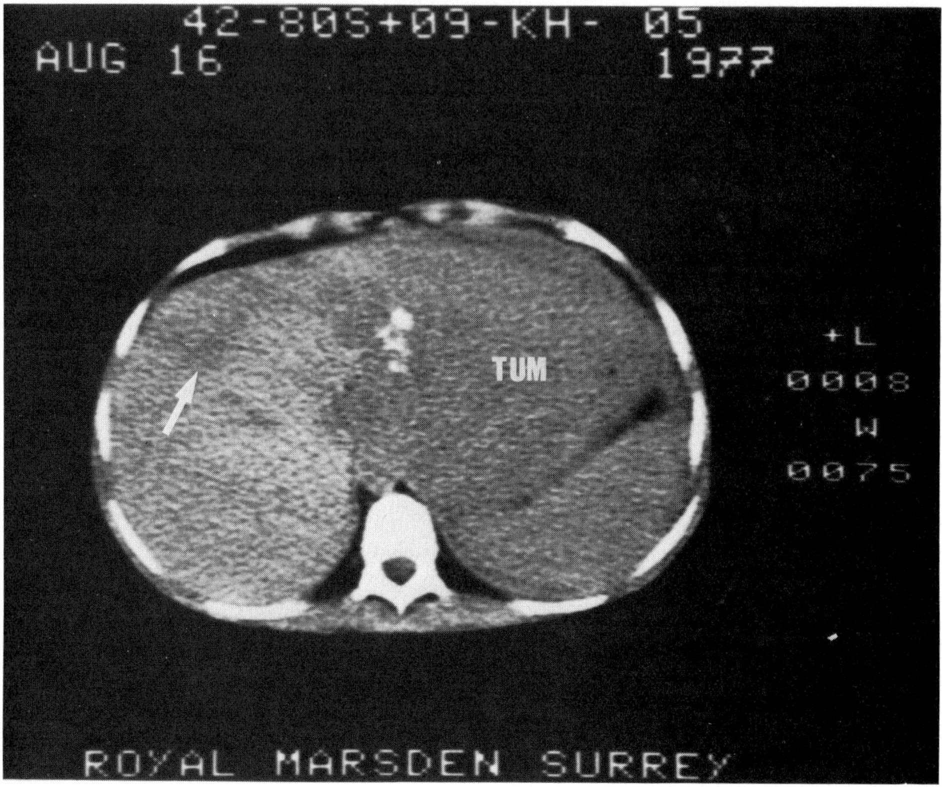

FIGURE 5. Hepatoma occupying left lobe (TUM). The tumor has a lower density than normal liver and contains calcification. Metastases in right lobe (arrow).

diffuse liver enlargement, which is easily identified with CT. The attenuation value may be close to that of normal liver[25] or significantly lower.[8] Figure 5 shows a large hepatoma occupying the left lobe with metastases in the right lobe. The density of the main tumor mass in the left lobe was lower than that of the surrounding liver parenchyma and did enhance after the administration of intravenous contrast material. Opacification is probably related to vascularity, the dose of iodine given, and the time interval between administration and the scan.[5] CT may also reveal unsuspected metastases in other parts of the liver as in Figure 5, or in adjacent lymph nodes (Figure 6). These findings were confirmed at laparotomy.

The ultrasound appearances of a primary hepatoma range from highly echogenic tumors—presumably due to high vascularity—to apparently cystic masses,[26] and we have seen examples at both ends of this spectrum.

Both ultrasound and CT, however, are useful noninvasive techniques for surveying the liver in patients suspected of having a primary hepatic neoplasm. Those with a history of cirrhosis, hemochromatosis, viral hepatitis,

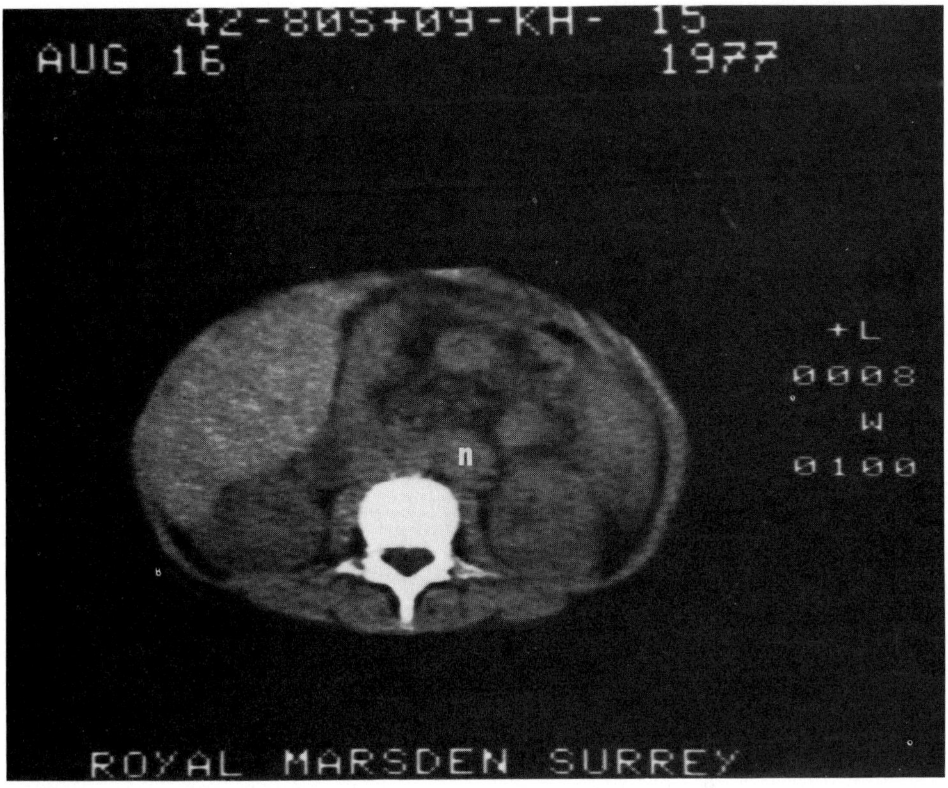

FIGURE 6. Para-aortic lymph node enlargement (n) in primary hepatoma (same patient as in Figure 5).

alcoholism or vinyl chloride exposure[27] are particularly at risk. These techniques may also be helpful in defining operability if radical surgery is considered, and in monitoring response to chemotherapy.

Although metastases are shown by both ultrasound and CT, the variety of appearances is much greater with ultrasound, and there is also a loose correlation between the ultrasound appearance and tumor type. The vast majority of metastases appear as low-density lesions with CT, whereas at least six different patterns have been described with ultrasound.[23]

Multiple metastases frequently vary in size and shape; these features are particularly well demonstrated with CT (Figure 7). Tumors as small as 2 cm in diameter usually can be identified, but lesions smaller than this may cause difficulty in identification. Even in retrospect, we were unable to detect metastases of 2 to 4 mm in diameter in the liver of a patient with pancreatic carcinoma. The lower the attenuation values, the smaller the lesion that can be recognized.[5] Intravenous contrast agents may be used to increase the density of normal liver tissue; simple manipulation of the window settings is

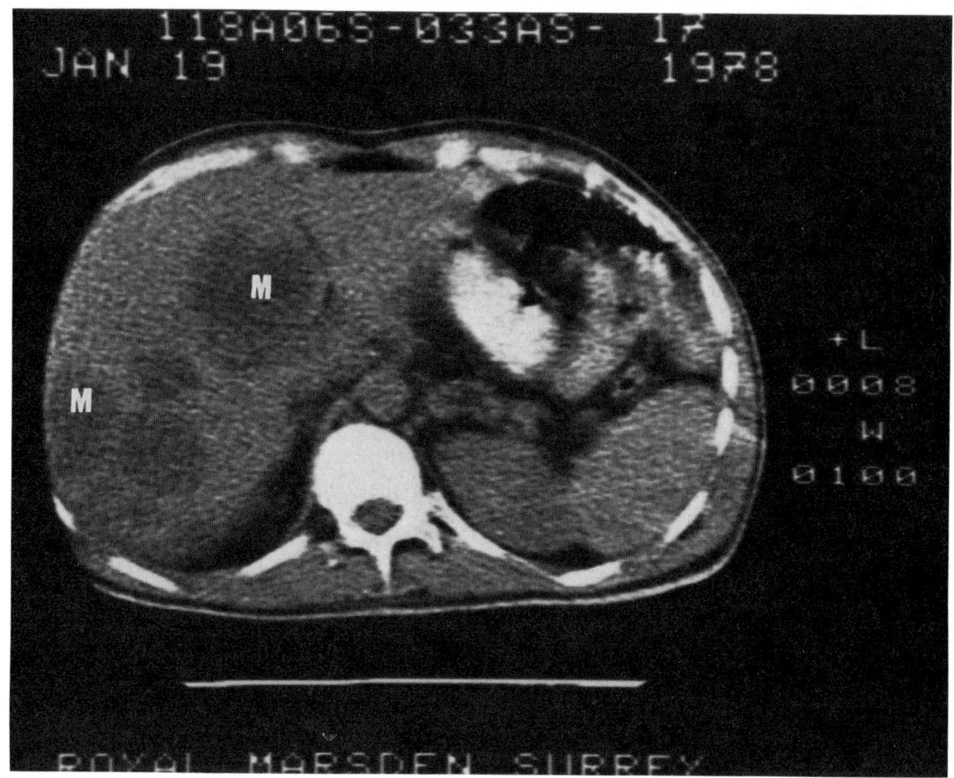

FIGURE 7. Multiple metastases in the liver (M).

also helpful in identifying suspicious deposits. Metastases containing calcium are clearly identified.[28] These arise from osteogenic sarcoma, colloid carcinoma of the colon and tumors of the ovary. Occasionally a metastasis contains an area of very low density in the center (0 to 5 Hounsfield units). This probably represents central necrosis within an avascular lesion. Metastases must be distinguished from other areas of low density which may be seen within the liver, namely portal vein branches and dilated intrahepatic bile ducts. This is not usually a problem in the periphery of the liver, where dilated bile ducts and normal vessels are too small to be identified. Difficulty may arise, however, near the liver hilum and in the left lobe, where dilated ducts and portal veins reach the size of 1 to 2 cm in diameter, and may be seen as rounded oval structures of diminished density. They tend to be more uniform in size and shape than metastases and have a more clearly defined edge.[29] Contrast enhancement may be helpful in distinguishing a space-occupying lesion from portal venous structures, since the latter become less obvious or completely disappear after contrast has been given. However, certain metastases have a high vascular element and are likely to opacify after

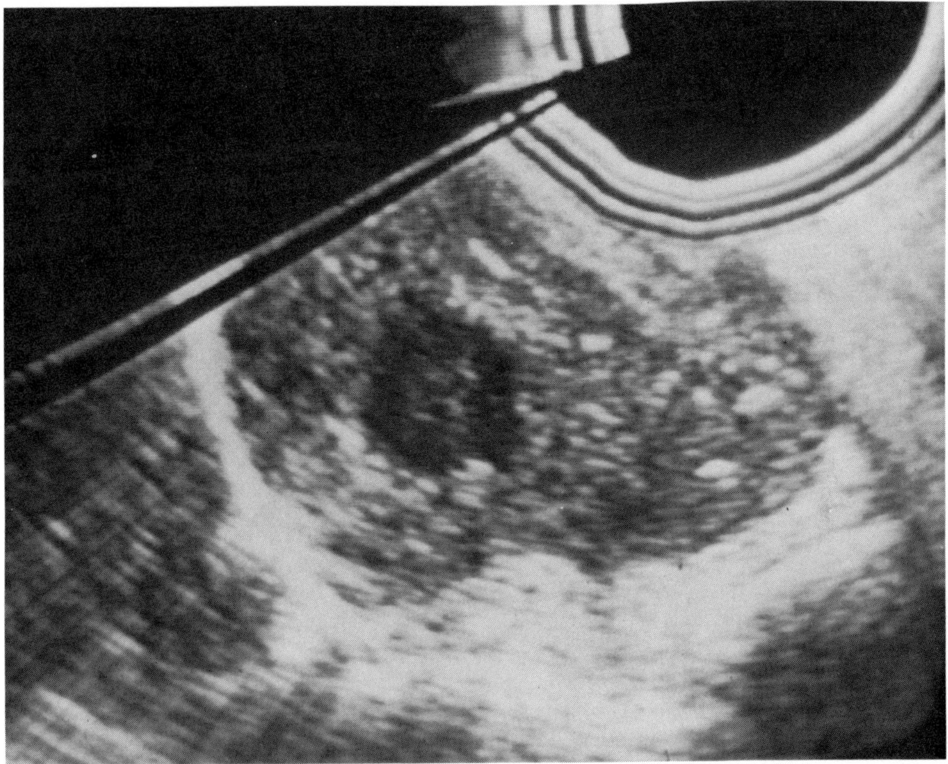

FIGURE 8. Metastasis in right lobe of liver returning echoes of lower amplitude than normal liver.

administration of contrast. These include metastases from endocrine tumors, renal carcinoma and melanoma.[30] It may, therefore, be impossible to exclude a small metastasis in the central part of the liver; and where suspicion is high, regular follow-up is essential.

With ultrasound, the majority of hepatic metastases seen in our department have echo amplitudes below those of normal liver (Figure 8), but this probably represents the effects of patient selection more than the normal distribution of appearances in the population as a whole. Clinics with a high proportion of gastrointestinal lesions may have a preponderance of echogenic lesions. In our experience, metastases from carcinoma of the colon and other intra-abdominal adenocarcinomas generally return high echo amplitudes (Figure 9). Occasionally, metastases reflecting both high and low amplitude echoes, are present in the same patient. Possible explanations for this anomaly are the difference in vascularity between the deposits, the presence of hemorrhage or necrosis, or secretion of mucin by some metastases. "Target" lesions have also been described with ultrasound (Figure 10). The significance of these types of deposit is uncertain but, again, the difference in

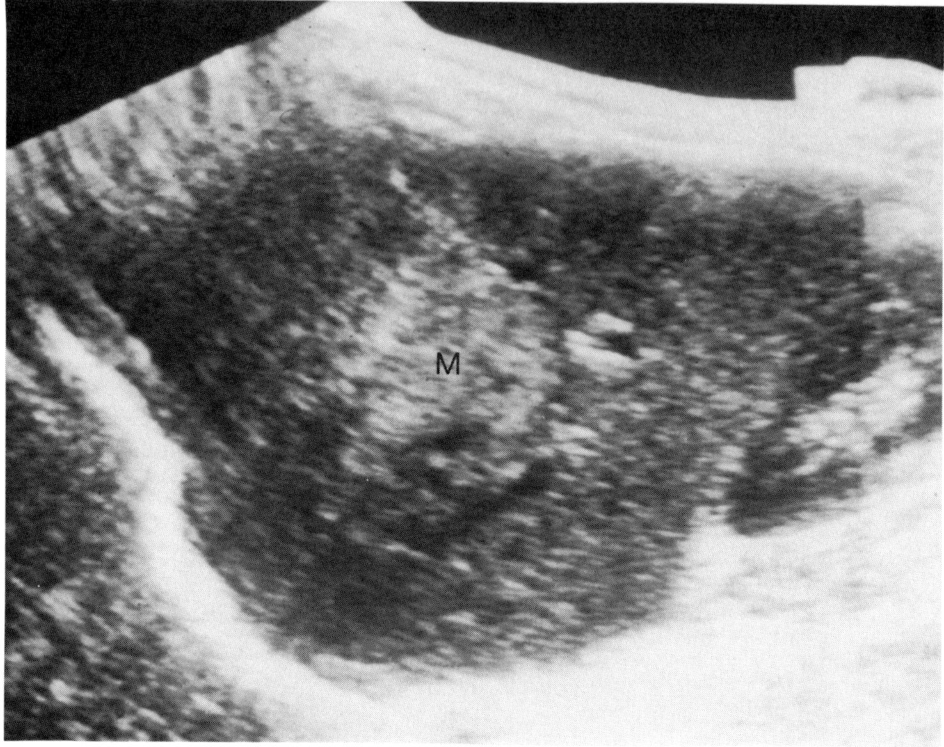

FIGURE 9. An "echogenic" metastasis (M) from carcinoma of the colon. Despite prior knowledge of its presence, this lesion could not be detected at CT scanning.

echo pattern in the center of the lesion may reflect hemorrhage or necrosis. Cystic metastases may sometimes be detected with ultrasound, but the walls of these lesions are usually thick and irregular in contrast to benign cysts, which have thin, smooth walls. This type of metastasis was commonly encountered by Taylor[19] in patients with carcinoma of the breast, but has not been seen by us in this disease, though we have seen them from kidney tumors and cystadenocarcinoma of ovary or pancreas.

Finally, metastases may reflect an echo amplitude similar to that of normal liver. In these circumstances, the metastasis is not identifiable. The incidence of this type of lesion is probably between 3 and 5 percent of tumors, and is similar to the situation with computed tomography, where the difference in density between the metastasis and normal liver is insufficient to allow detection. Although the exact incidence of this problem with both techniques is as yet uncertain, we have not seen a patient with proven metastases where both techniques were negative. To date, however, CT has had a somewhat higher incidence of false negative results than ultrasound.

Since ultrasound shows intrahepatic vessels more clearly than CT, there is little difficulty in distinguishing them from space-occupying lesions; in ad-

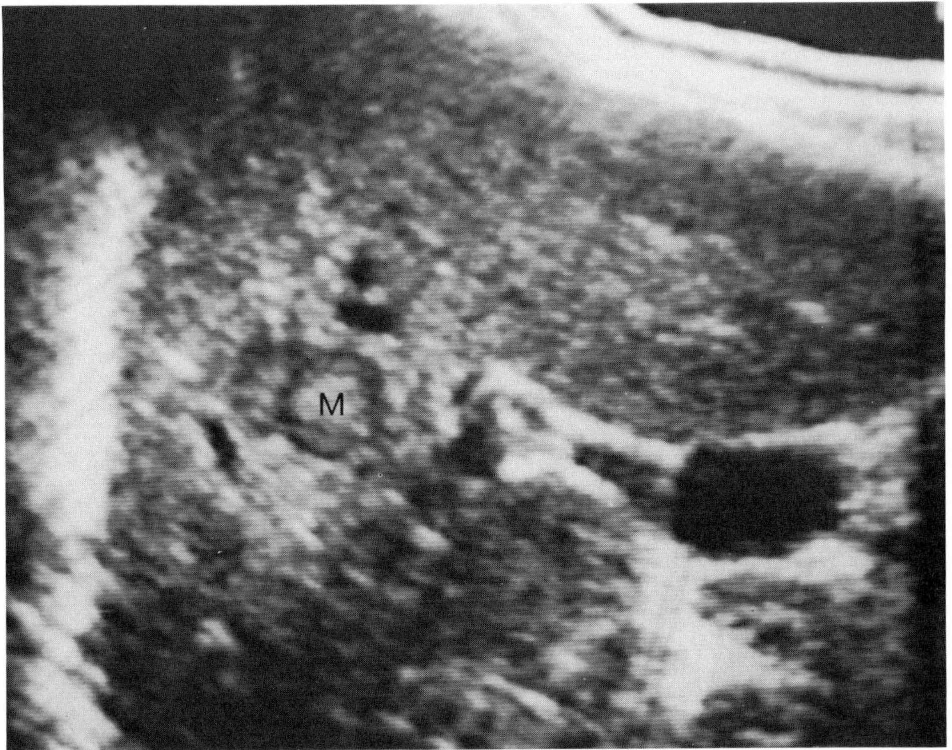

FIGURE 10. One form of "target" metastasis (M) in the liver.

dition, the ultrasound scanner can be steered into the plane of the long axis of the vessel to confirm its connection with the portal vein or inferior vena cava (Figure 2). As with CT, normal-sized intrahepatic bile ducts are not shown but are readily recognised when dilated.[31] The walls of these ducts are easily identified and they do not, therefore, cause a problem in the differential diagnosis of metastases. A diagnostic accuracy of 96.5 percent has been reported in the use of ultrasound to distinguish hepatocellular jaundice from extrahepatic obstruction.[32]

Benign Tumors

Benign tumors are rare and, again, our experience is necessarily limited. Figure 11 shows a CT scan of a patient with a benign hepatic cell adenoma. The density is significantly lower than that of normal liver tissue, and there is no enhancement after the administration of intravenous contrast medium. Sagel, Stanley and Evens[33] also reported the CT appearances of an hepatic adenoma with central necrosis, confirmed at surgery. There was normal en-

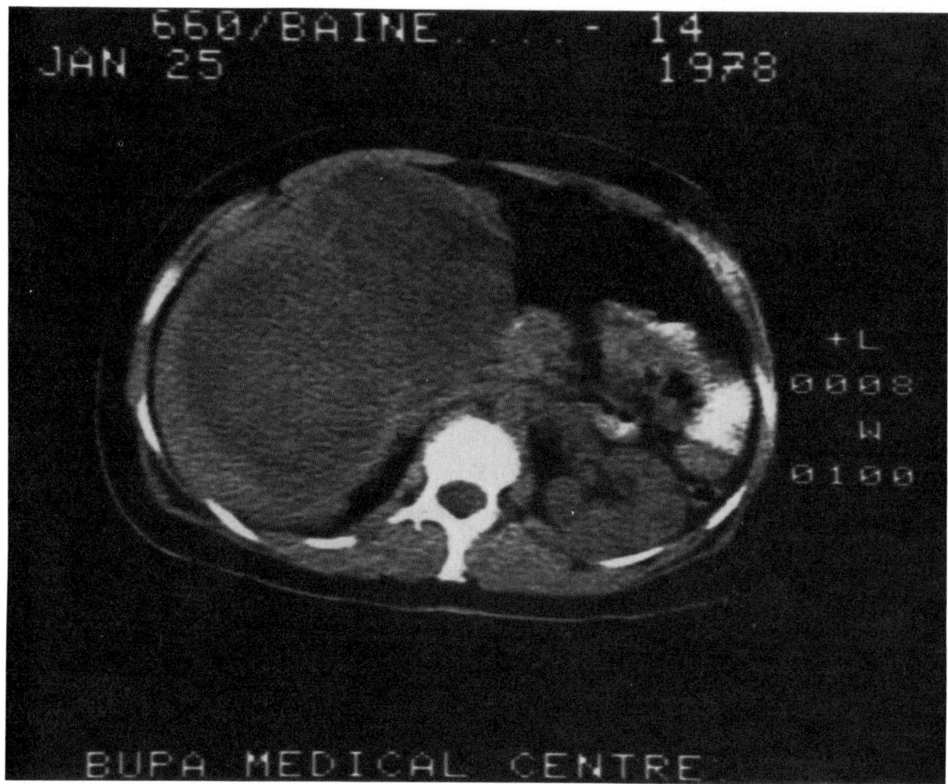

FIGURE 11. Benign hepatic adenoma. A large low-density lesion is shown in the right lobe of the liver. (Printed by kind permission of the BUPA Medical Centre).

hancement of the periphery, but the central part of the tumor did not opacify. Stephens et al[34] have reported a cavernous hemangioma of the liver which did enhance after contrast. Clearly CT findings in benign tumors are not specific, and depend upon vascularity, degree of necrosis and other factors affecting attenuation values which have previously been discussed.

The ultrasound findings in benign hepatic adenoma are those of a complex mass, often with multiple cystic spaces. Although unusual, we cannot yet say how specific this appearance is for this disorder.

Both capillary, venous, and arteriovenous malformation may occur in the liver and can be recognised on ultrasonic scanning. Capillary lesions are seen as clearly defined echogenic masses which may be indistinguishable from echogenic metastases (Figure 12). However, they are almost invariably solitary and do not change in size and shape with time. They may occasionally calcify and cause acoustic shadowing.

Lesions containing larger vessels may appear as complex, small, multicystic masses and have a rather characteristic appearance which we have not

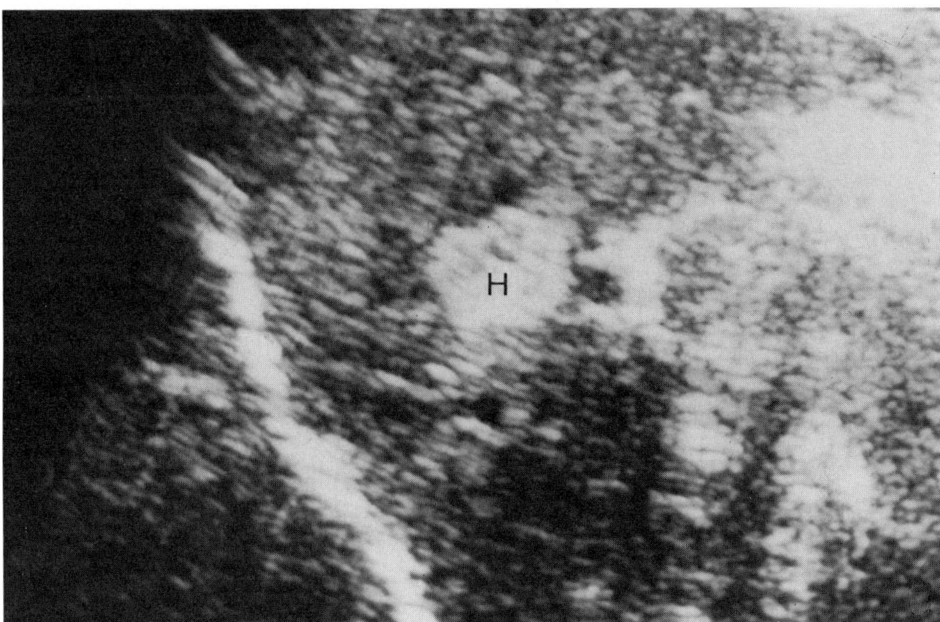

FIGURE 12. A capillary hemangioma of the liver (H). Note the clearly defined border.

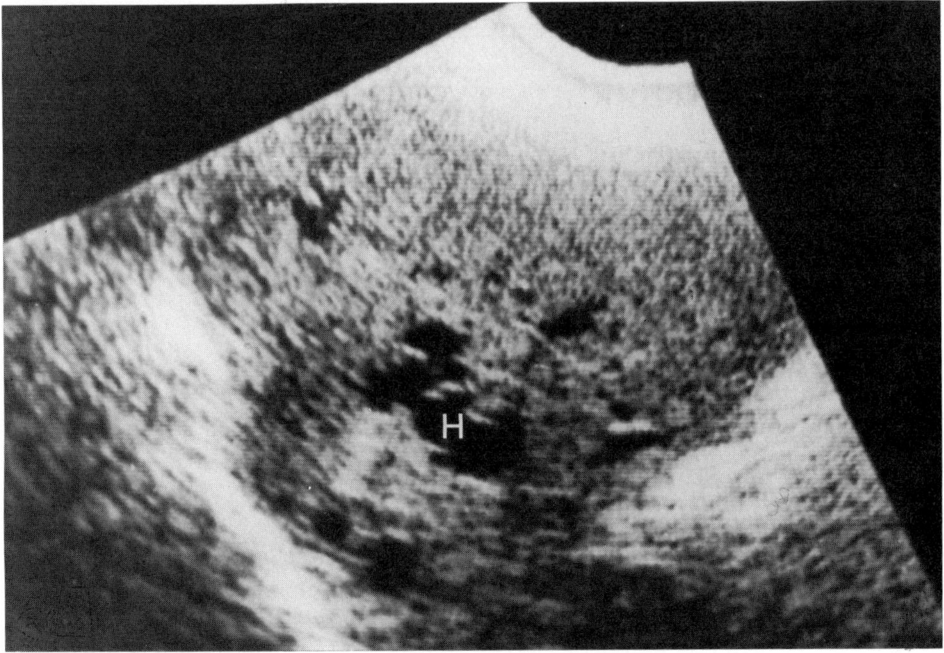

FIGURE 13. A venous hemangioma (H) in the right lobe of the liver. (Kindly supplied by Dr. K. Dewbury, Southampton).

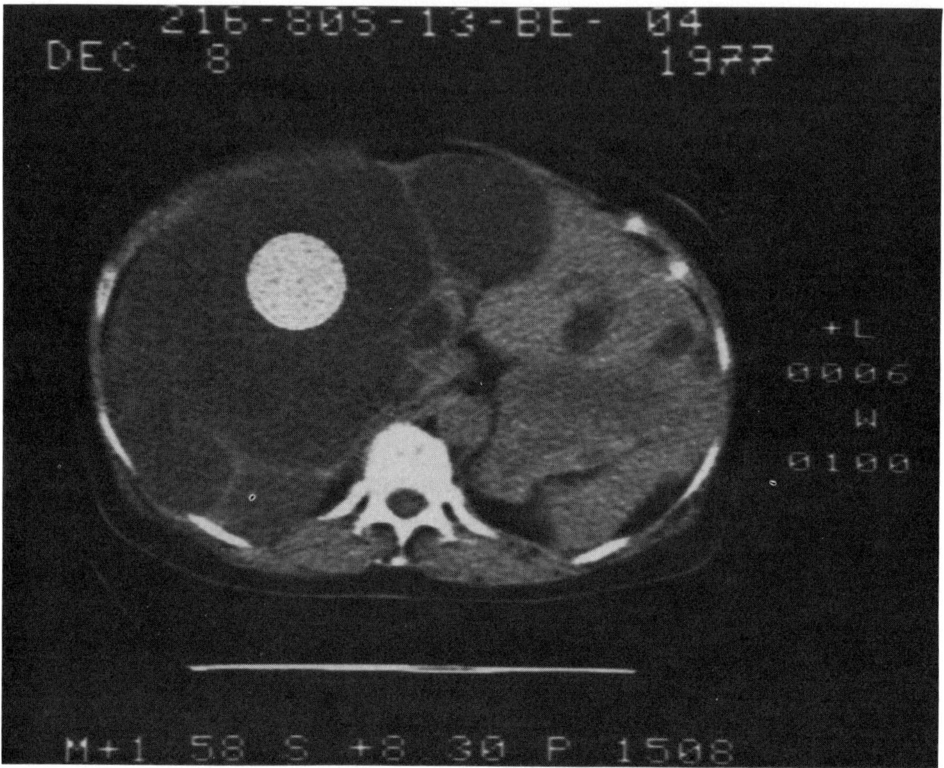

FIGURE 14. Benign hepatic cysts occupying the major part of the right lobe. The density of the lesion has been measured within the "region of interest" shown by the white disk. Mean value = 1.58 EMI units; S D ± 8.30.

seen mimicked by other types of abnormality (Figure 13). Ultrasound has the advantage over CT that it is possible to define the internal structure of these benign masses.

Cysts

Both CT and ultrasound are able to distinguish cysts from solid tumors, and there is a high degree of accuracy with ultrasound.[35] The accuracy of CT requires further evaluation and there are as yet few reports in the world literature. Levitt et al[12] diagnosed 6 cysts in a group of 266 patients. Two were proved correct and the remaining four were thought to be correct in view of the subsequent clinical course. Using CT, the attenuation values are close to that of water (approximately 0 to 10 Hounsfield units); with ultrasound a cyst is echo-free. Ultrasound also clearly demonstrates a well defined thin wall. The wall of the cyst is not shown with CT as it has a density similar to that of normal liver parenchyma (Figure 14). The edge of the lesion, however, is usually well defined in contrast to the edge of a mestastasis, which is irregular and ill defined. A cyst may be affected by partial volume averaging with

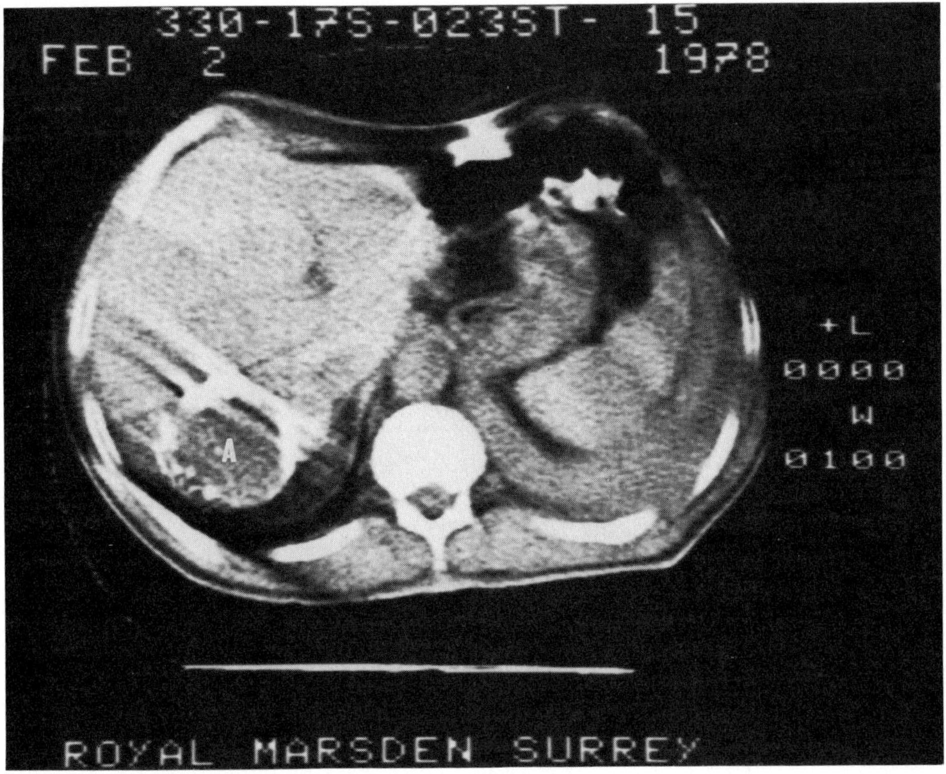

FIGURE 15. Chronic amebic abscess (A). There is dense calcification within the wall, which has produced streak artifacts.

both CT and ultrasound. Falsely high readings for attenuation values, or an echo pattern within the cyst, may therefore be obtained. If the lesion is smaller than 2 cm in diameter, it may then be difficult to distinguish from a solid tumor.

Hydatid cysts are infrequently seen in the United Kingdom, but the ultrasound appearances are usually characteristic: they may be multiple; they usually have a thicker, more laminated wall than simple cysts; and daughter cysts may be seen within the main lesion. There may also be a thin layer of calcification within the walls; this is clearly shown with CT, and is the main criterion by which a hydatid cyst is differentiated from a simple one. Occasionally, however, hydatid cysts have an appearance both with ultrasound and CT which is indistinguishable from a benign simple cyst.

Abscesses

A liver abscess can usually be recognised with both CT and ultrasound, but it may be difficult to reach a definitive diagnosis on the scan appearances alone. With CT, the attenuation values characteristically fall between those of

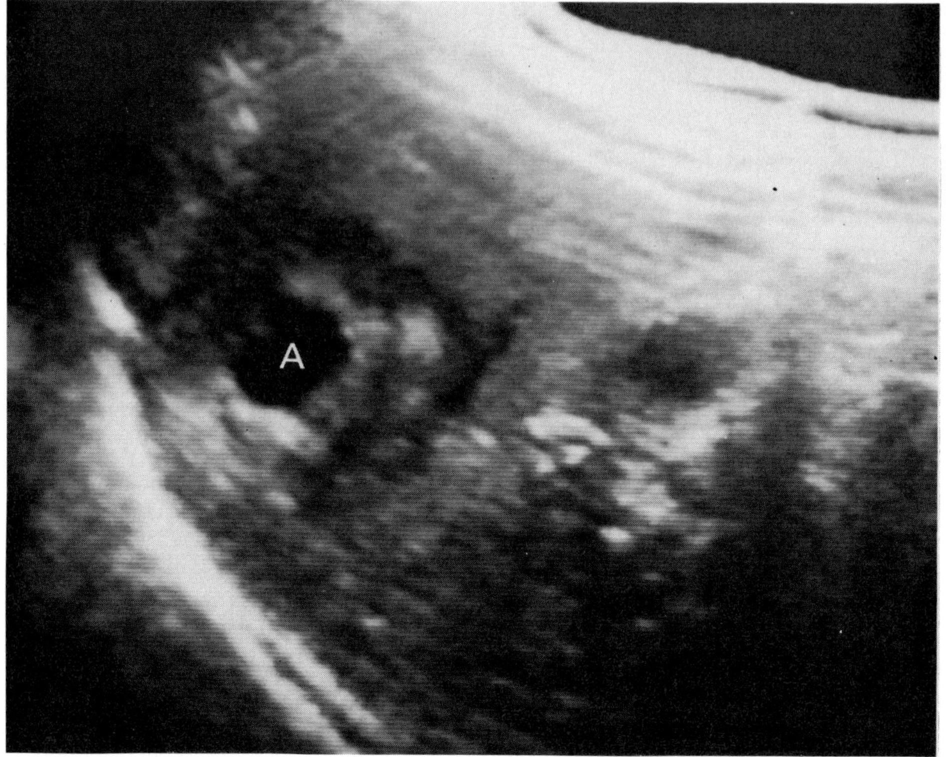

FIGURE 16. An hepatic abscess (A) high in the right lobe.

a cyst and those of a neoplasm.[12] However, if the attenuation values fall close to those of a cyst (0 to 10 Hounsfield units) or neoplasm (10 to 15 Hounsfield units below normal liver) then the correct diagnosis cannot be made reliably with CT. The clinical history of the patient usually clarifies the situation.

A chronic amebic abscess (Figure 15) may contain calcification. The attenuation values within the lesion in this patient are similar to those of normal liver parenchyma.

Using ultrasound, differentiation between a cyst and an abscess is generally easier, as an abscess tends to have a thick, irregular wall, and necrotic debris can usually be seen within[36, 37] (Figure 16). Occasionally, this may form a characteristic fluid level. Problems with ultrasound do arise in distinguishing an abscess from a cystic metastasis or a necrotic metastasis, both of which cannot be reliably differentiated on the ultrasound appearances alone.

Subphrenic Abscess

A collection of fluid between the diaphragm and liver can usually be detected by both techniques, but CT is probably more reliable, especially for left-sided lesions. A right subphrenic abscess produces a characteristic appearance with CT: the liver edge is compressed medially, forming a rather straight border. The density of the lesion is lower than that of normal liver parenchyma. A subphrenic abscess must be distinguished from ascites, which surrounds not only the liver but also the spleen. Both CT and ultrasound can be used to guide needle biopsy or aspiration.[38, 39]

Differential Diagnosis

It is generally easier to reach a narrower differential diagnosis with ultrasound than with CT, since each pathological process tends to have a more specific appearance on ultrasound scanning.

The scan findings must always be interpreted with reference to the patient's history and clinical findings.

Lesions in organs adjacent to the liver may compress and alter its contour. This is particularly true of lesions in the right kidney and suprarenal gland.[11] The isotope scan, or indeed the ultrasound examination, may indicate a lesion to be in the right lobe of the liver when it is, in fact, in an adjacent organ. The layer of fat between the right lobe of the liver and kidney is seldom disturbed even by large renal tumors, and is extremely useful in determining the origin of such a mass on CT scans.

Conclusions

We have attempted to define the capabilities and limitations of ultrasound and computed tomography in the evaluation of focal liver disease. It is clear that these techniques have an advantage over isotope scanning since both provide information regarding the composition of a lesion. Although isotope techniques can detect lesions as small as 3 cm in diameter, differential diagnosis of the "cold area" is not possible.[40] Furthermore, lesions in other organs, for example the right kidney, may compress the liver edge and be interpreted on the isotope scan as originating in the right lobe of the liver. However, radionuclide hepatic imaging is simple, carries a low morbidity and is relatively cheap. The diagnostic accuracy in detecting a space-occupying lesion is high and it is therefore likely to remain a very useful initial screening test. A recent study by Grossman et al[41] indicates that radionuclide imaging, computed tomography and ultrasound are all complementary. In a group of 50 patients, a combination of ultrasound and gamma imaging identified all lesions, whereas CT alone or in combination with ultrasound or radionuclide imaging was, in certain instances, unsuccessful.

It is clear that ultrasound and CT give similar information, but since they rely on completely different physical characteristics, the disadvantages of one system are frequently balanced by the advantages of the other. For example, ultrasound is often unsuccessful in the obese patient; the CT scan is not only unaffected by adipose tissue, but is easier to interpret. Conversely, very thin patients are ideal ultrasound subjects, but their lack of intra-abdominal fat may result in poor organ demarcation on CT. It is important to attempt to assess the relationship of ultrasound and CT in terms of relevant clinical information provided. In our view, both procedures will be able to detect the lesion and provide information regarding its nature in the majority of instances. It is usually unnecessary to subject the patient to two different types of examination. Ultrasound is much cheaper than CT, quicker to perform, and easily repeatable. For these reasons, it is almost certainly the first investigation which should be undertaken for the detection of focal liver disease, and it is especially suited to follow-up examinations. Ultrasound is also particularly valuable as a screening test for the presence of metastases in patients undergoing surgery for primary malignant tumors. It would be quite impractical to use CT in this way as it is only possible to perform a limited number of CT examinations per day. In view of all these factors, we consider that CT should be reserved for those patients in whom liver ultrasound has been unsuccessful, or where there is some difficultly in interpretation. The number of patients then referred for CT would clearly depend upon the expertise of the ultrasonographer. It is also important to emphasize that not all centers at present have both ultrasound and CT equipment available.

Future developments are likely to improve spatial resolution in both ultrasound and CT. Ultrasound equipment will probably become more automatic, resulting in less dependence upon operator expertise. Further technical developments, especially in the field of signal analysis, will eventually permit more accurate recognition of different tissues and possibly, ultimately, non-invasive "biopsy".

References

1. Hounsfield GN: Computerized transverse axial scanning (tomography): (1) description of system. Br J Radiol 46:1016–1022, 1973.
2. Hill KR: The EMI scanner: technical aspects. Br J Hosp Med—Equipment Supplement 11:5–14, 1974.
3. Wells PNT: Resolution in pulse-echo system. In: Ultrasonics in Clinical Diagnosis, ed. Wells PNT, Edinburgh, Churchill Livingstone, 1977.
4. Taylor KJW, Carpenter DA, Hill CR, McCready VR: Grey scale ultrasound imaging: the anatomy and pathology of the liver. Radiology 119:415–423,1976.
5. Stephens DH, Sheedy PF, Hattery R, MacCarty R: Computed tomography of the liver. Am J Roentgenol 128:579–590, 1977.
6. Harell GS, Marshall WH, Breiman RS, Seppi EJ: Early experience with the varian six second body scanner in the diagnosis of hepatobiliary tract disease. Radiology 123. 335–360, 1977.
7. McCullough EC, Payne JT, Baker HL Jr, Hattery RR, Sheedy PF, Stephens DH, Gedgaudus E: Performance evaluation and quality assurance of computed tomography scanners, with illustrations from the EMI, ACTA and Delta scanners. Radiology 120:173–188, 1976.

8. Alfidi RJ, MacIntrye WJ, Haaga JR: The effects of biological motion on CT resolution. Am J Roentgenol 127:11–15, 1976.
9. Taylor KJW, Hill CR: Scanning techniques in grey scale ultrasonography. Br J Radiol 48: 918–920, 1975.
10. Meire HB, Farrant P: Preparation of the patient for abdominal ultrasound scanning. Br J Radiol 51:387–388, 1978.
11. Kreel L: Computerized tomography using the EMI general purpose scanner. Br J Radiol 50:2–14, 1977.
12. Levitt RG, Sagel SS, Stanley RJ, Jost RG: Accuracy of computed tomography of the liver and biliary tract. Radiology 124(1):123–128, 1977.
13. Carlsen EN, Filly RA: Newer ultrasonographic anatomy in the upper abdomen: I. The portal and hepatic venous anatomy. J Clin Ultrasound 4:85–96, 1976.
14. Sample WF: Techniques for improved delineation of normal anatomy of the upper abdomen and high retroperitoneum with grey scale ultrasound. Radiology 124:197–202, 1977.
15. Mategrano MD, Petasnick J, Clark J, Chung Bin A, Weinstein R: Attenuation values in computed tomography of the abdomen. Radiology 125:135–140, 1977.
16. New PFJ, Aronow S: Attenuation measurements of whole blood and blood fractions in computed tomography. Radiology 121:635–640, 1976.
17. Stanley R, Sagel SS, Levitt R: Computed tomography of the body: early trends in application and accuracy of the method. Am J Roentgenol 127:53–67, 1976.
18. Alfidi RJ, Haaga JR, Havrilla TR, Pepe RG, Cook SA: Computed tomography of the liver. Am J Roentgenol 127:69–74, 1976.
19. Taylor KJW: Ultrasonic investigation of the hepatobiliary system and spleen. In: Ultrasonics in Clinical Diagnosis, ed. Wells PNT, Edinburgh, Churchill Livingstone, 1977.
20. Alfidi RJ, Haaga JR, Meaney TF, MacIntyre WJ, Gonzales L, Tarar R, Zelch MG, Boller M, Cook SA, Jelden G: Computed tomography of the thorax and abdomen: a preliminary report. Radiology 117:257–264, 1975.
21. Taylor KJW: The liver. In: Atlas of Gray Scale Ultrasonography, ed. Taylor KJW, Edinburgh, Churchill Livingstone, 1978.
22. Scheible W, Gosink BB, Leopold GR: Echographic patterns of hepatic metastatic disease. In: Ultrasound in Medicine, ed. White D, New York, Plenum Press, 3A:463–464, 1977.
23. Meire HB: Grey scale echographic appearances of liver metastases. In: Ultrasound in Medicine, ed. White D, New York, Plenum Press, 3A:315–319, 1977.
24. Petasnick JP, Clark JW: Computed tomography of the abdomen: initial experience. Gastrointest Radiol 1:201–208, 1976.
25. Sheedy PF, Stephens DH, Hattery RR, Muhm JR, Hartman GW: Computed tomography of the body: initial clinical trial with the EMI prototype. Am J Roentgenol 127:23–51, 1976.
26. Green B, Bree RL, Goldstein HM, Stanley C: Grey scale ultrasound evaluation of hepatic neoplasms: patterns and correlations. Radiology 124:203–208, 1977.
27. Williams DMJ, Smith PM, Taylor KJW, Crossley IR, Duck BW: Monitoring liver disorders in vinyl chloride monomer workers using grey scale ultrasonography. Br J Indust Med 33:152–157, 1976.
28. Kreel L: Computerized tomography of the liver. Clin Radiol 28:571–581, 1977.
29. Kressel HY, Korobkin M, Goldberg HI, Moss AA: The portal venous tree simulating dilated biliary ducts on computed tomography of the liver. J Computor Assisted Tomography 1(2):169–175, 1977.
30. Viamonte M Jr, Schiff E: Diagnostic approach to hepatic malignant neoplasms. JAMA 238 (20):2191–2193, 1977.

31. Husband JE, Meire HB, Kreel L: Comparison of ultrasound and computor-assisted tomography in pancreatic diagnosis. Br J Radiol 50:855–862, 1977.

32. Taylor KJW, Rosenfield AT: Grey-scale ultrasonography in the differential diagnosis of jaundice. Arch Surg 112:820–825, 1977.

33. Sagel SS, Stanley RJ, Evens RG: Early clinical experience with motionless whole-body computed tomography. Radiology 119:321–330, 1976.

34. Stephens DH, Hattery RR, Sheedy PF: Computed tomography of the abdomen: early experience with the EMI body scanner. Radiology 119: 331–335, 1976.

35. Pollack HM, Goldberg BB: Kidney. In: Abdominal Grey-Scale Ultrasonography, ed. Goldberg BB, New York, Wiley, 1977.

36. Albertson KW, Leopold GR: Liver. In: Abdominal Grey-Scale Ultrasonography, ed. Goldberg BB, New York, Wiley, 1977.

37. Taylor KJW, McCready VR: A clinical evaluation of grey scale ultrasonography. Br J Radiol 49:244–252, 1976.

38. Haaga JR, Alfidi RJ: Precise biopsy localization by computed tomography. Radiology 118:603–607, 1976.

39. Smith EH, Bartrum RJ: Ultrasonically guided percutaneous aspiration of abscesses. Am J Roentgenol Radium Ther Nucl Med 122:308, 1974.

40. McCready VR: Scintigraphic studies of space-occupying liver disease. Sem Nucl Med 2(2):108–127, 1972.

41. Grossman ZD, Wistow BW, Bryan PJ, Dinn WM, McAfee JG, Kieffer SA: Radionuclide imaging, computed tomography and grey-scale ultrasonography of the liver: a comparative study. J Nucl Med 18:327–332, 1977.

Complementary Use of Ultrasound and Isotope Scanning of the Liver

DANIEL SULLIVAN

Radionuclide imaging of the liver has been a useful tool for many years, but does not always provide the degree of clinical certainty which most physicians desire. For this reason, ultrasonic and computerized tomographic imaging of the liver are of major interest. Since each technique contributes certain unique information, and since none of the methods is clearly superior to the others, interactive applications have become popular. However, there are few good comparative studies, and currently accepted practices are often based largely on anecdotal experiences, institutional preferences, and personal bias. In this paper, the complementary uses of scintigraphy and ultrasound are reviewed. The role of computerized tomography is discussed elsewhere in this issue.

Hepatic scintigraphy is a standardized procedure which can be reproducibly performed on all patients. There are no significant adverse effects, and the radiation burden is low. The examination reflects abnormality in hepatic function as well as in structure, and it gives an overview of the entire liver and spleen.

Nevertheless, some features of hepatic scintigraphy are frustrating. The reliable in vivo resolution is approximately 2 cm, although lesions less than 1 cm can occasionally be detected with optimum equipment and technique. The findings on radioisotope liver studies are seldom characteristic of a specific etiologic diagnosis, and further tests are often necessary. The extensive overlap of normal and abnormal appearances gives rise to a relatively high incidence of false positive and equivocal readings.[1-4] Studies of liver scintigraphy performed during the past ten years have reported accuracy ranging from 70 to 90 percent; an overall accuracy of approximately 85 percent is typi-

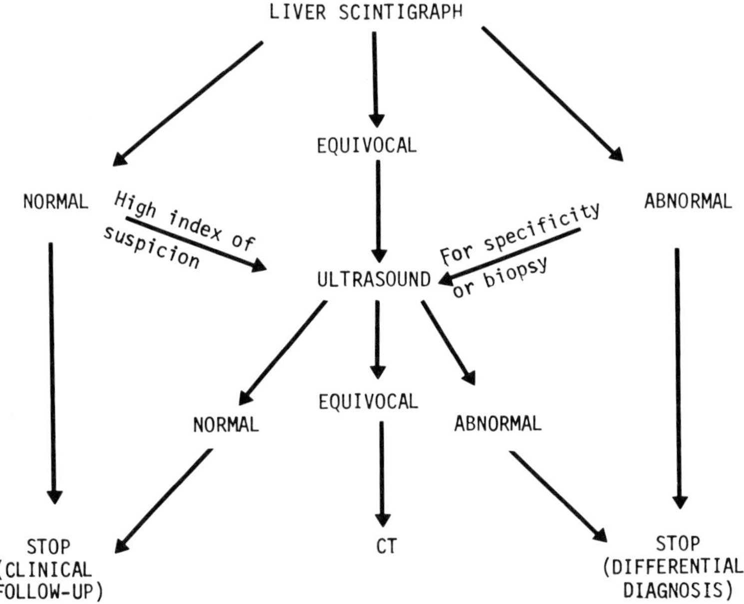

FIGURE 1. Decision tree for hepatic imaging. Current integration of noninvasive methods.

cal.[5-12] Despite these limitations, scintigraphy is acceptable for screening purposes and more useful than other single tests.

Ultrasound examination is not routinely used as a screening procedure for several reasons: the technique is tomographic and often must be adapted to the individual patient; the reproducibility of sonographic results is inconsistent because quality is highly dependent upon operator ability; occasionally, parts of the liver are acoustically inaccessible owing to gas, ribs, bandages, scar, or colostomy.

On the other hand, the resolution of ultrasound is usually less than 1 cm. The echotomograms display sectional anatomy, internal organ structure, and tissue consistency. The sonographic appearances may indicate a specific diagnosis in many cases. The accuracy of gray-scale liver ultrasound scanning ranges from 80 to 94 percent in the few reported studies.[3, 13-19] Because of the great variation in technical quality of ultrasound images, it is not yet possible to predict the levels of accuracy, sensitivity, and specificity which might be consistently achieved.

We believe that scintigraphy is, in most cases, the appropriate initial imaging technique for detecting abnormal hepatic morphology. The role of ultrasound depends then, as illustrated in Figure 1, on the outcome of the radionuclide study.

If the scintigraph is normal, should the patient be studied with ultrasound? In most cases, no. The purpose of ultrasound examination would be to detect lesions in those patients with false negative scintigraphs. False neg-

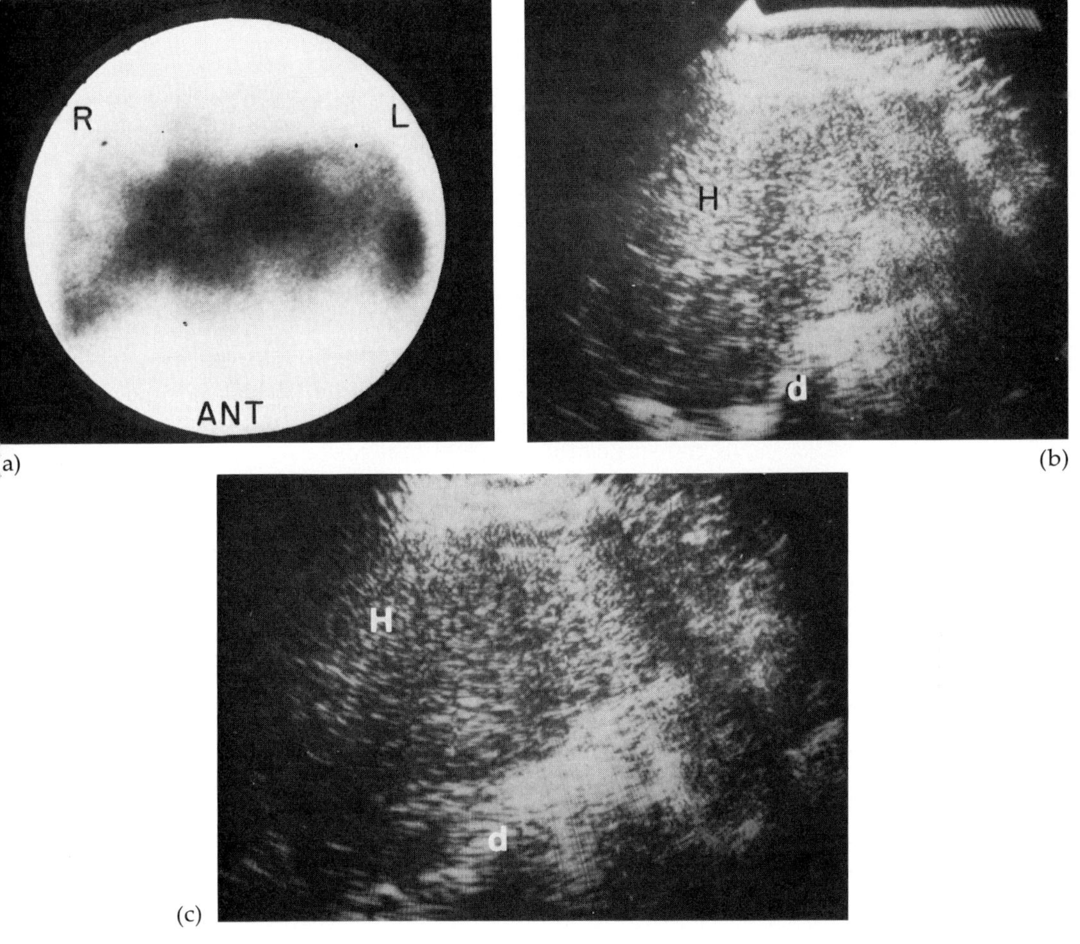

(a) (b) (c)

FIGURE 2. (a) Anterior scintigraph from a 60 year-old man with adenocarcinoma of the colon. There are multiple areas of decreased activity consistent with extensive metastatic disease. This was confirmed by follow-up studies (H = liver; d = diaphragm).

(b and c) Ultrasound examination done on the same day as the scintigraph in Figure 2a detected no abnormalities. Two representative oblique echotomograms are shown.

ative scintigraphs are usually due to early diffuse disease or small, scattered lesions. In theory and in practice, such lesions are also difficult to detect with ultrasound, and there are no data yet to indicate that ultrasound will detect those lesions in a significant number of patients.

Figure 2 illustrates this problem. The patient has proven hepatic metastases from colon adenocarcinoma. The scintigraph shows obvious disease, but the ultrasound examination performed on the same day appears normal. A repeat ultrasound study done a few days later with careful attention to technique and TGC (time gain compensation) settings suggested heterogeneous areas in the liver, but the findings were not striking.

At least three factors can contribute to detection problems. One is lateral resolution. Superimposed echoes from laterally adjacent structures or normal parenchyma can obscure small lesions or narrow bands of infiltrative disease. A second factor is the tomographic process. Small, scattered lesions between tomographic planes can be missed. A third factor is the acoustic nature of the lesion. If the abnormal tissue is more sonolucent or sonodense than normal liver, the probability of detection is higher. If the lesion is acoustically similar to normal tissue, then recognition will be difficult.

The true incidence of these false negative ultrasound results is not known. Careful attention to echographic technique is essential to minimize such errors. Good quality, gray-scale equipment must be used, and the technologist must have adequate training and experience in optimum adjustment of TGC controls. In addition, to detect subtle parenchymal disease, we believe that the white-on-black display is preferable to the black-on-white format, which floods the retina with background illumination.

Certainly, if there is strong clinical suspicion of liver abnormality despite normal scintigraphy, then ultrasound examination is justified. In particular, preliminary studies suggest that ultrasound may produce fewer false negatives than scintigraphy in the detection of breast metastases, lymphoma, and fatty infiltration.[3, 16, 20] If these studies are confirmed, routine hepatic ultrasound in breast tumor and lymphoma patients will be a welcome clinical tool.

If the scintigraphic results are equivocal, should the patient be referred for ultrasonography? We performed a prospective study to answer this question. A group of 100 patients with equivocal scintigraphs had directed ultrasound examinations of the equivocal areas, and were followed clinically to obtain a proven diagnosis.[17] The overall accuracy of the scintigraphic interpretations of "probably normal" and "probably abnormal" was only 74 percent. The directed ultrasound studies correctly identified normality and abnormality in 93 percent of the cases. On the basis of this study, we have adopted the procedure of automatically and routinely proceeding to directed ultrasound examination when the liver scintigraph is equivocal.

To the question, "Why not start with ultrasound, if the accuracy is higher?" we answer that our ultrasonographer knew the scintigraphic results and gave maximum attention to the area in question. Several investigators agree with our belief that directing the ultrasound examination in this way enhances its utility and accuracy. We do not yet know whether the excellent results achieved by isotopically directed ultrasound studies can be extrapolated to ultrasonic imaging as a primary screening test.

In our study, ultrasound was particularly useful in differentiating normality from abnormality when the equivocal finding was a relatively localized area. For example, sonography was highly accurate in evaluating suspected edge lesions, suspected lesions in the porta hepatis, suspected lesions in the gallbladder or renal fossae, and suspected lesions in the normal, but thin, left lobe. Figure 3 shows the utility of ultrasound in evaluating the portal region

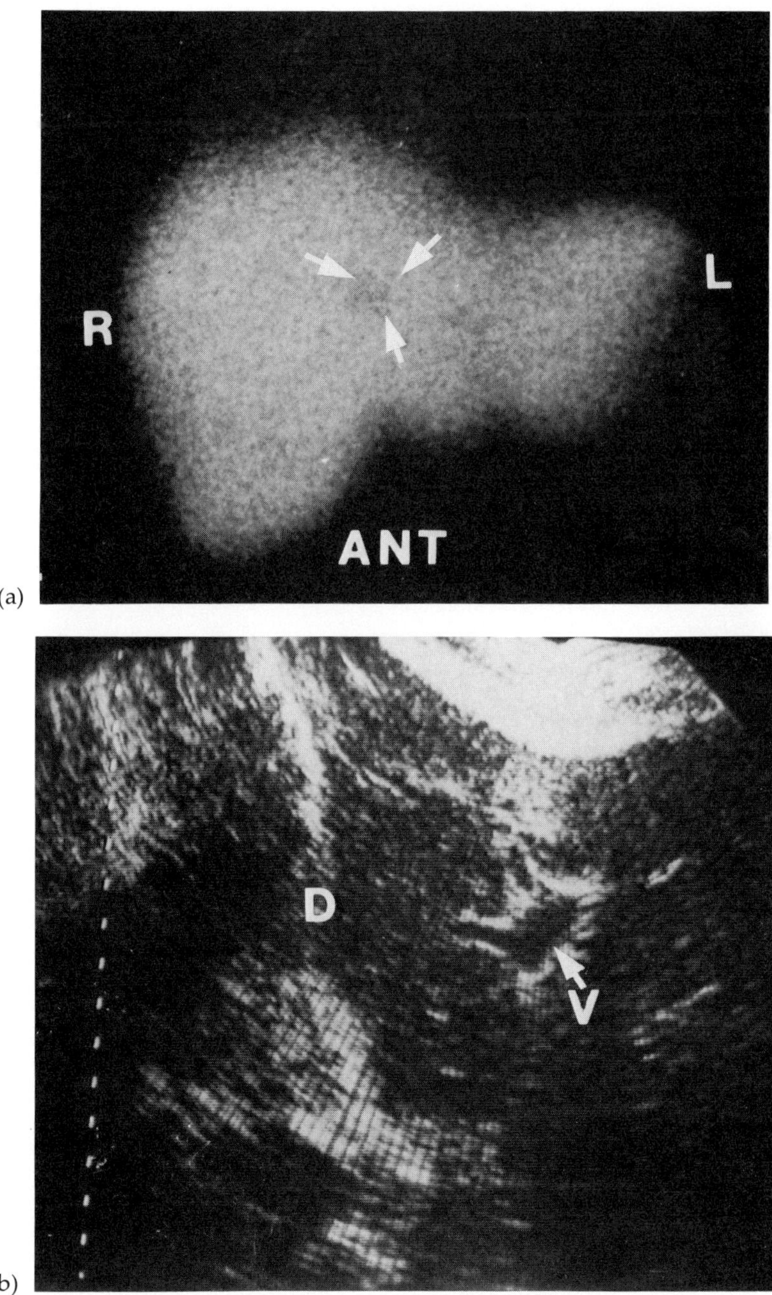

FIGURE 3. (a) Anterior scintigraph from a 66 year-old man being evaluated for weight loss. A questionable focal defect is present (arrows).

(b) Sagittal sonogram through the equivocal area. A normal, but prominent, venous confluence (V) is responsible for the "cold" defect on the scintigraph. The patient was followed clinically for six months and no primary or secondary tumor was found. (D = diaphragm).

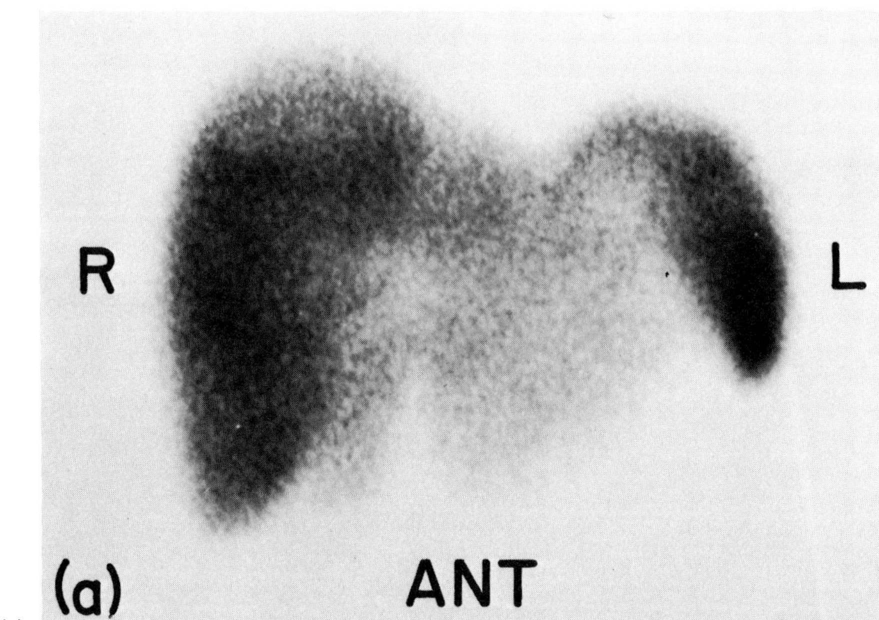

(a)

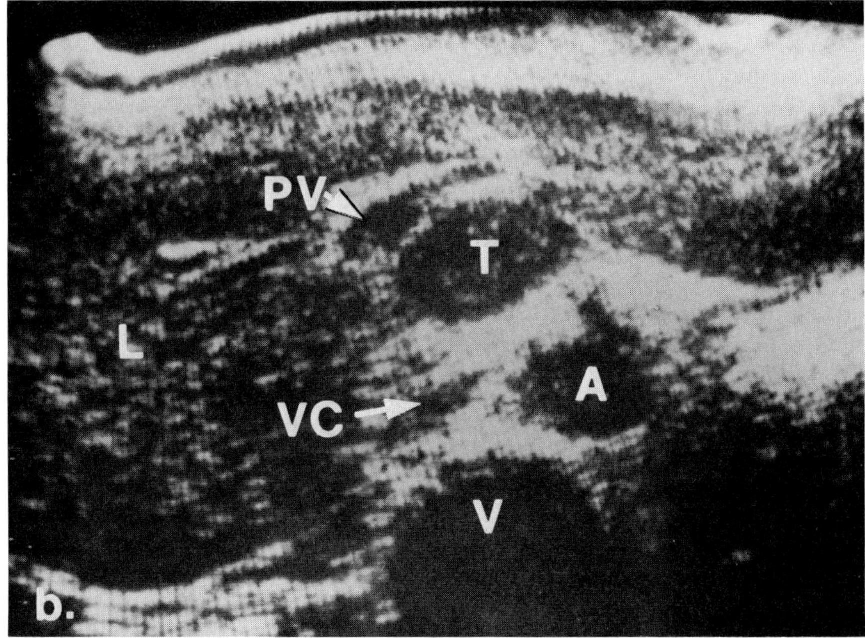

(b)

FIGURE 4. (a) Anterior scintigraph from a 65 year-old woman with lymphoma. The region of the porta hepatis is slightly prominent, suggesting the possibility of a mass.

(b) Transverse echotomogram showing tumor mass (T) bowing the splenic vein anteriorly at its transition into the portal vein (PV). (L = liver; VC = inferior vena cava; A = aorta; V = vertebral column).

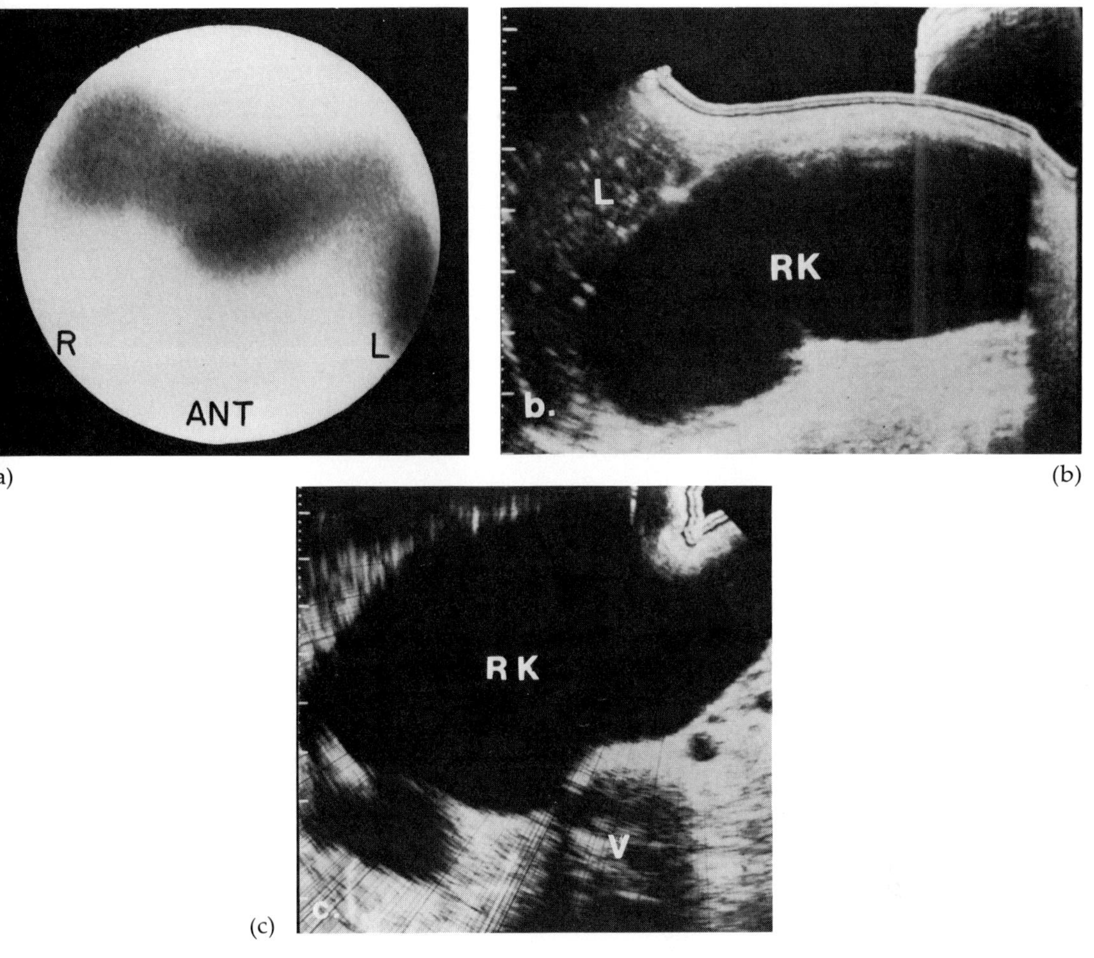

FIGURE 5. (a) Anterior scintigraph from a 24 year-old man. The possibility of hepatomegaly had been raised on a routine physical examination. The radioisotope study shows a small right lobe and suggests that the palpable mass is extrinsic to the liver.

(b and c) Sagittal and transverse sections from the ultrasound study, showing a large cystic lesion replacing the right kidney (RK) and presenting directly beneath the anterior abdominal wall. Surgery revealed massive hydronephrosis secondary to congenital uretero-pelvic obstruction (L = liver; V = vertebral column).

when scintigraphy is indeterminate; Figure 4 illustrates the value of sonography for investigating questionable focal lesions in the liver parenchyma; and Figure 5 is a case in which ultrasound clarified the nature of an edge lesion.

When the equivocal finding was diffuse inhomogeneity, ultrasound was also generally accurate in distinguishing normality from abnormality. The hepatic metastases shown in Figure 6 produced only questionable patchiness on the isotope study, but were clearly demonstrated by ultrasound (contrast this adenocarcinoma with the one shown in Figure 2, which was not acousti-

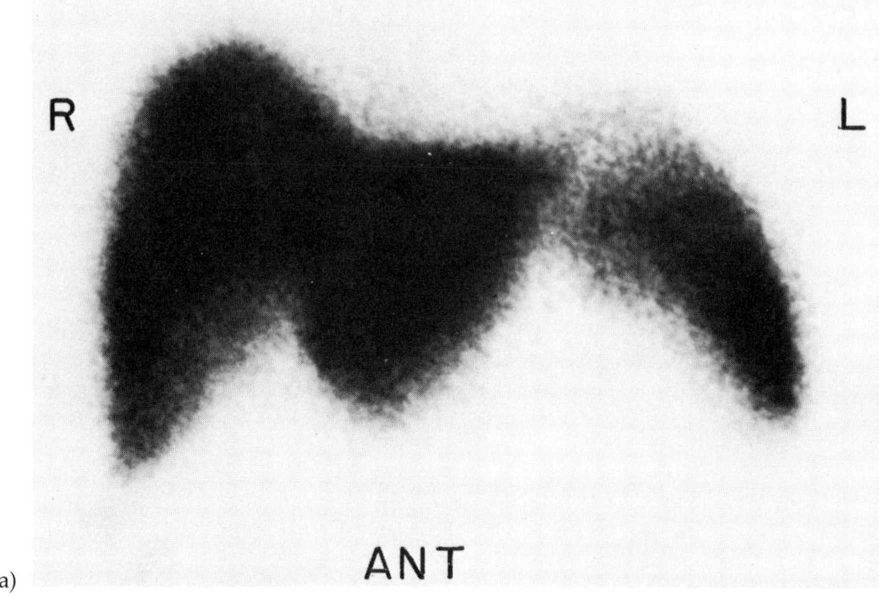

(a)

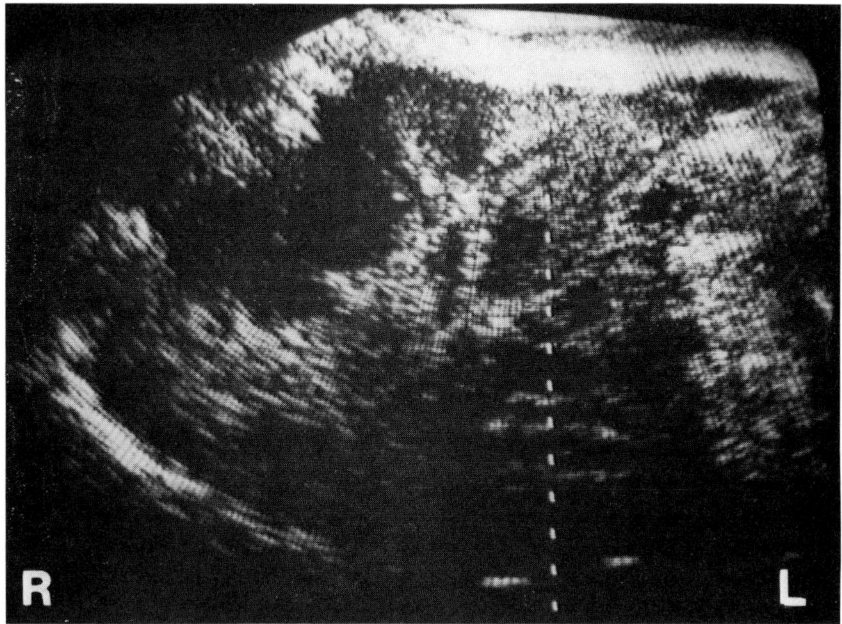

(b)

FIGURE 6. (a) Anterior scintigraph from a 56 year-old woman with right upper quadrant pain. The distribution of activity is nonhomogeneous but there are no discrete focal defects.

(b) Transverse echotomogram from the same patient shows large, irregular, echolucent areas replacing much of the liver parenchyma. Metastatic adenocarcinoma from an unknown primary site was found at laparotomy.

cally resolved. Further investigation into the relationship between histologic differences and sound transmission will undoubtedly lead to improved accuracy and specificity for ultrasound examination). However, as discussed above, the accuracy of ultrasound was decreased in this group by difficulty with some cases of diffuse disease or small lesions.

When the results of sonographic and scintigraphic examinations are discordant, on which study should the physician rely? In our study of 100 patients, the combination of a "probably normal" scintigram and an abnormal echogram never occurred. The combination of a "probably abnormal" scintigram and a normal echogram occurred 15 times. Ultrasound was correct in 14 (93 percent) of these cases; that is, the scintigraphic result was almost always a false positive. Based on these data, we believe that the ultrasound result is most likely to be correct in discordant cases. However, more data are needed, and if there is clinical doubt about the validity of the ultrasound result, further evaluation is warranted (see Figure 2).

Multiplane tomographic scintiscanners have been developed, and some investigators advocate their use in evaluating equivocal liver scintigraphs.[21, 22] At the present time, however, ultrasound seems to be more useful than the multiplane nuclear scanners for liver imaging.

If the scintigraph is definitely abnormal, should ultrasound examination be done? In many cases, a constellation of characteristic scintigraphic abnormalities which coincides with the clinical findings makes further tests unnecessary. For example, multiple focal lesions in a patient with suspected metastatic disease may be sufficiently specific to be diagnostic. In other cases, the scintigraphic findings may be compatible with several diagnoses such as cyst, abscess, or tumor; or they may be most consistent with a diagnosis that is not consonant with the clinical setting. There are several radionuclide techniques which can be used to narrow the differential diagnosis of the nonspecific defects seen on colloid scintigraphs. These ancillary procedures include gallium scans and blood pool studies (both dynamic and static). Although these techniques are helpful, ultrasound examination often provides more diagnostic specificity.[19, 23-27] For example, we have seen patients with known extrahepatic tumors in whom a solitary focal defect on scintigraphy was found by ultrasound to be a benign cyst rather than a metastatic tumor.

Furthermore, if needle biopsy of a lesion seen on an isotope study is desired, ultrasound is a relatively easy, noninvasive and effective method of localization. Thus, when the scintigraph is abnormal, ultrasound should be performed (a) if the scintigraphic findings are at variance with the clinical picture, or (b) if sonographic characterization of the nonspecific findings is desired—in particular, to determine cystic vs solid consistency.

There are certain clinical settings in which a sequence different from that discussed above might be preferred. For example, ultrasound examination is often ordered initially in patients who present with a palpable abdominal mass. However, if the mass is in the upper abdomen, potentially involving the liver or spleen, we advocate radionuclide examination in conjunction

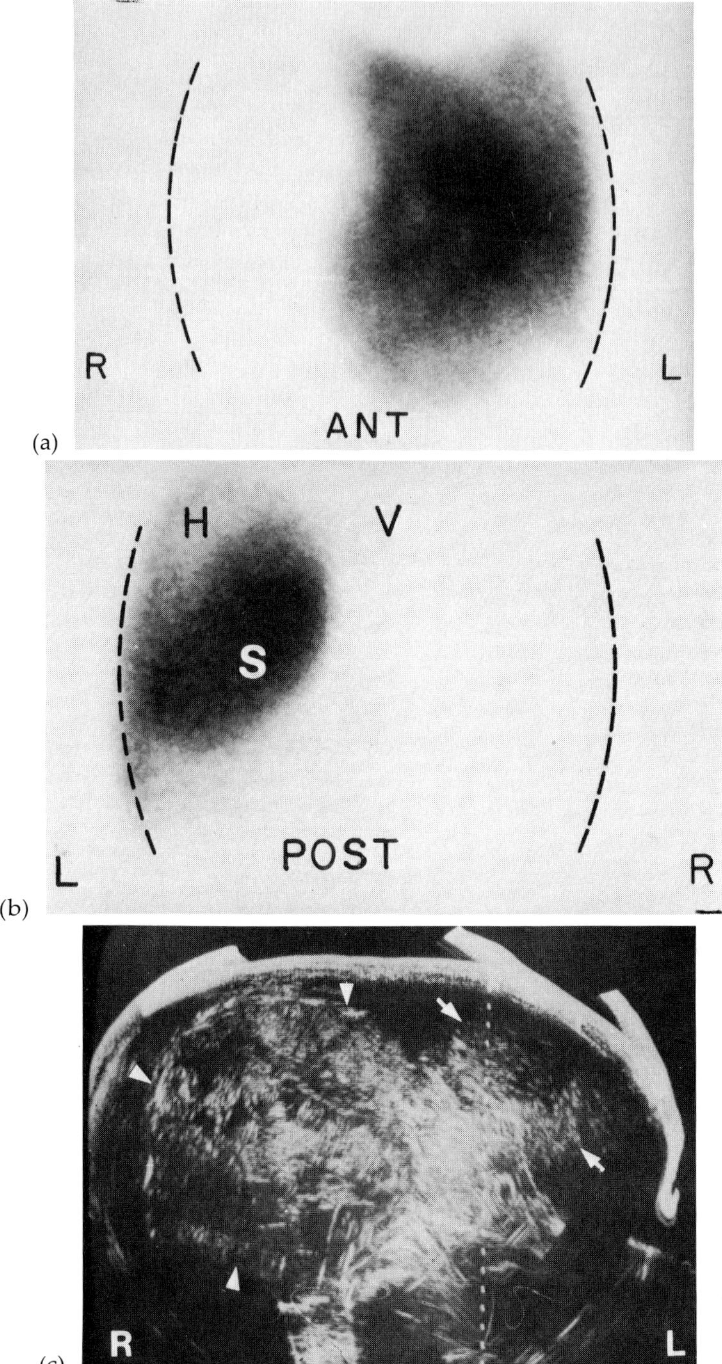

FIGURE 7. (a and b) Anterior and posterior views from liver scintigraphy in a 24 year-old woman with an upper abdominal mass. The dotted lines correspond to the patient's flanks. The liver is pushed anteriorly and to the left by an extrinsic right upper quadrant mass (H = liver; S = spleen; V = vertebral column).

(c) Transverse echotomogram done prior to the scintigraph. Structure in right upper quadrant (arrowheads) was interpreted as liver with diffuse metastases. Scintigraph suggested, and autopsy confirmed, that the right upper quadrant mass was entirely tumor and the left upper quadrant structure (arrows) was the liver.

with ultrasonography. A prior scintigraph is analogous to a scout film before radiographic tomography—a road map that will assist the technologist in obtaining the most pertinent information, and will aid the physician in interpreting the results. Figure 7 shows an unusual, but dramatic, example of the value of such an overview. The patient was a 24 year-old woman who presented acutely with a large, painful abdominal mass. An emergency ultrasound examination correctly diagnosed this as hemorrhage into a malignant tumor, but misinterpreted the scan as diffuse tumor of the liver. The scintigraphs, done soon after, demonstrated that the liver was actually displaced from the right upper quadrant by some extrinsic mass. Autopsy revealed a massive hypernephroma of the right kidney pushing the liver into the left upper quadrant. There was no tumor in the liver. The area thought to be diseased liver on ultrasound was the primary tumor itself—an error which might have been avoided had the scintigraphic "scout film" been available to the ultrasonographer.

Patients with suspected intrahepatic or parahepatic abscesses are often referred initially for ultrasound. This is appropriate because the specificity, sensitivity, and accuracy of ultrasound in the diagnosis of abscess, especially in or around the liver, is over 90 percent.[28] Nevertheless, scintigraphy is often helpful in conjunction with ultrasound (a) to confirm the sonographic findings and (b) to evaluate the entire liver and spleen.

Patients who are jaundiced should be studied initially by ultrasound. The reliability of ultrasound in detecting biliary distension is greater than 95 percent; thus, the etiology of the jaundice as intrahepatic vs extrahepatic may be determined.[29] The status of the liver parenchyma, porta hepatis, gallbladder and pancreas can be evaluated at the same time. Scintigraphy plays a secondary role in these patients, despite the development of ^{99m}Tc-labeled hepatobiliary agents.[30] These new radiopharmaceuticals produce superior images compared to the more familiar ^{131}I-rose bengal. However, the inherent resolution limitations of contemporary gamma cameras make it unlikely that these studies can equal or surpass the ability of ultrasound to display bile ducts and gallstones. These agents will be useful in demonstrating functional aspects of the hepatobiliary system, such as cystic duct patency, and could be complementary to ultrasound in certain situations. For example, ultrasound is reliable in detecting gallstones but cannot make the distinction between acute and chronic cholecystitis. Preliminary investigations with ^{99m}Tc-labeled hepatobiliary agents (cholescintigraphy) have shown that visualization (filling) of the gallbladder excludes acute cholecystitis and that nonvisualization (non-filling) of the gallbladder is virtually specific for acute cholecystitis.[31] The routine clinical utility of these studies needs further elaboration.

The ability of ultrasound to clearly delineate cystic structures makes sonography particularly useful in patients with suspected choledochal cysts or Caroli's disease. Since turnover of cyst contents may be too slow to allow accumulation of radiopharmaceutical, hepatobiliary scintigraphy is only occasionally helpful. However, the functional information, if obtainable, is valuable in some cases.

The protocol presented here exploits the strengths of both modalities.

Some of the interactions may differ slightly at other institutions because of legitimate differences in equipment and expertise. Further technological advances in imaging will undoubtedly change the relative efficacies in at least some, if not all, of these applications. However, the decision tree shown in Figure 1 represents the most accurate and cost effective approach for detecting abnormal hepatic morphology at the present time.

References

1. Covington E: Pitfalls in liver photoscans. Am J Roentgenol 109:745, 1970.
2. Freeman L, Meng C, Johnson P, Bernstein R, Bosniak M: False positive liver scans caused by disease processes in adjacent organs and structures. Br J Radiol 42:651, 1969.
3. Johnson P, Sweeney W: The false-positive hepatic scan. J Nucl Med 8:451, 1967.
4. McClelland R: Focal porta hepatis scintiscan defects: what is their significance? J Nucl Med 16:1007, 1975.
5. Cedermark B, Schultz S, Bakshi S, Parthasarathy K, Mittelman A, Evans J: The value of liver scan in the follow-up study of patients with adenocarcinoma of the colon and rectum. Surg Gynec Obstet 144:745, 1977.
6. Fee H, Prokop E, Cameron J, Wagner H: Liver scanning in patients with suspected abdominal tumor. JAMA 230:1675, 1974.
7. Lunia S, Parthasarathy K, Bakshi S, Bender M: An evaluation of sulfur colloid liver scintiscans and their usefulness in metastatic workup. J Nucl Med 16:62, 1975.
8. McCready V: Scintigraphic studies of space-occupying liver disease. Semin Nucl Med 2: 108, 1972.
9. Nilsson T, Edeling C, Lavaetz O, Munck O, Olsen T: Predictive value of liver scintiphotography for demonstration of metastases in malignant gastrointestinal disorders. Acta Chir Scand 142:231, 1976.
10. Oster Z, Larson S, Strauss H, Wagner H: Analysis of liver scanning in a general hospital. J Nucl Med 16:450, 1975.
11. Read D, Hambrick E, Abcarian H, Levine H: The preoperative diagnosis of hepatic metastases in cases of colorectal carcinoma. Dis Col Rect 20:101, 1977.
12. Ruiter D, Byck W, Pauwels E, Taconis W, Spaander P: Correlation of scintigraphy with short interval autopsy in malignant focal liver disease. Cancer 39:172, 1977.
13. Koch C, Pauwels E: Evaluation of ultrasonic and scintigraphic studies of the liver. Radiologia Clin 45:282, 1976.
14. Leyton B, Halpern S, Leopold G, Hagen S: Correlation of ultrasound and colloid scintiscan studies of the normal and diseased liver. J Nucl Med 14:27, 1973.
15. McArdle C: Ultrasonic diagnosis of liver metastases. J Clin Ultrasound 4:265, 1976.
16. Smith I, Taylor K, McCready V, Powles T, Bondy P: A comparison of grey-scale ultrasound with other methods for the detection of liver metastases from breast carcinoma. Clin Oncol 2:47, 1976.
17. Sullivan D, Taylor K, Gottschalk A: The use of ultrasound to enhance the diagnostic utility of the equivocal liver scintigraph. Radiology 128:727–732, 1978.
18. Taylor K, Carpenter D, Hill C, McCready, V: Grey-scale ultrasound imaging. Radiology 119:415, 1976.

19. Zatz L, Goulding J, Hanley G: A comparison of grey-scale ultrasound and radionuclide imaging for the detection of focal hepatic lesions: open shutter technique. J Clin Ultrasound 5:178, 1977.
20. Glees J, Taylor K, Gazet J, Peckham M, McCready V: Accuracy of grey-scale ultrasonography of liver and spleen in Hodgkin's disease and the other lymphomas compared with isotope scans. Clin Radiol 28:233, 1977.
21. Sample W: Correlative studies between multi-plane tomographic nuclear imaging and grey-scale ultrasound in extra and intrahepatic abnormalities. Ultrasound in Med 2:175, 1976.
22. Sample W, Gray R, Poe N: Nuclear imaging, tomographic nuclear imaging, and grey-scale ultrasound in the evaluation of the porta hepatis. Radiology 122:773, 1977.
23. Bryan P, Dinn W, Grossman Z, Wistow B, McAfee J, Kieffer S: Correlation of computed tomography, gray scale ultrasonography, and radionuclide imaging of the liver in detecting space-occupying processes. Radiology 124:387, 1977.
24. Garrett W, Kossoff G, Uren R, Carpenter D: Gray scale ultrasonic investigation of focal defects on ^{99m}Tc sulphur colloid liver scanning. Radiology 119:425, 1976.
25. Grossman Z, Wistow B, Bryan P, Dinn W, McAfee J, Kieffer S: Radionuclide imaging, computed tomography, and grey-scale ultrasonography of the liver: a comparative study. J Nucl Med 18:327, 1977.
26. Pritchard J, Winston M, Berger H, Blahd W: Diagnosis of focal hepatic lesions: combined radioisotope and ultrasound techniques. JAMA 229:1463, 1974.
27. Taylor K, Sullivan D, Rosenfield A, Gottschalk A: Grey-scale ultrasound and isotope scanning: complementary techniques for imaging the liver. Am J Roentgenol 128:277, 1977.
28. Taylor K, Wasson, JFMcI, DeGraaff C, Rosenfield A, Andriole V: Accuracy of grey-scale ultrasound diagnosis of abdominal and pelvic abscesses in 220 patients. Lancet 1:83, 1978.
29. Taylor K, Rosenfield A: Grey-scale ultrasonography in the differential diagnosis of jaundice. Arch Surg 112:820, 1977.
30. Ronai P: Hepatobiliary radiopharmaceuticals: defining their clinical role will be a galling experience. J Nucl Med 18:488, 1977.
31. Stadalnik R, Matolo N, Jansholt A, Krohn K, DeNardo G, Wolfman E: Technetium-99m pyridoxylideneglutamate (P.G.) cholescintigraphy. Radiology 121:657, 1976.

Normal Anatomy of the Pancreas by Computed Tomography and Diagnostic Ultrasound

JOSEPH F. SIMEONE
BRUCE D. SIMONDS

Computerized Tomography

The pancreas lies in the upper abdomen, with its tail very close to the hilum of the spleen. From this point the pancreas arches anteriorly in front of the upper pole of the left kidney and in front of the left adrenal gland (Figure 1). The body continues in the midline, located anterior to the superior mesenteric artery from which it is separated by low-density fat. After crossing the midline the organ turns posteriorly; the head is located in front of the inferior vena cava and below the caudate lobe of the liver. The second portion of the duodenum is located just lateral to the head. Inferior to the head and the body are the third and fourth portions of the duodenum, which pass posterior to the superior mesenteric vessels. The antrum of the stomach is located anterior to the head, and the body and fundus of the stomach are located in front of the body and the tail of the pancreas. The uncinate process is often seen just posterior to the superior mesenteric vessels (Figure 2). Very often the splenic vein can be seen as a separate structure just posterior to the body and tail of the pancreas, but as it approaches the superior mesenteric vein, these two veins usually blend imperceptibly with the normal density of the pancreas.[1]

In all but the thinnest patients, the pancreas is completely surrounded by fat that is of lower CT density than the pancreas. In very thin patients, dilute contrast material in the stomach and duodenum outlines the anterior margin

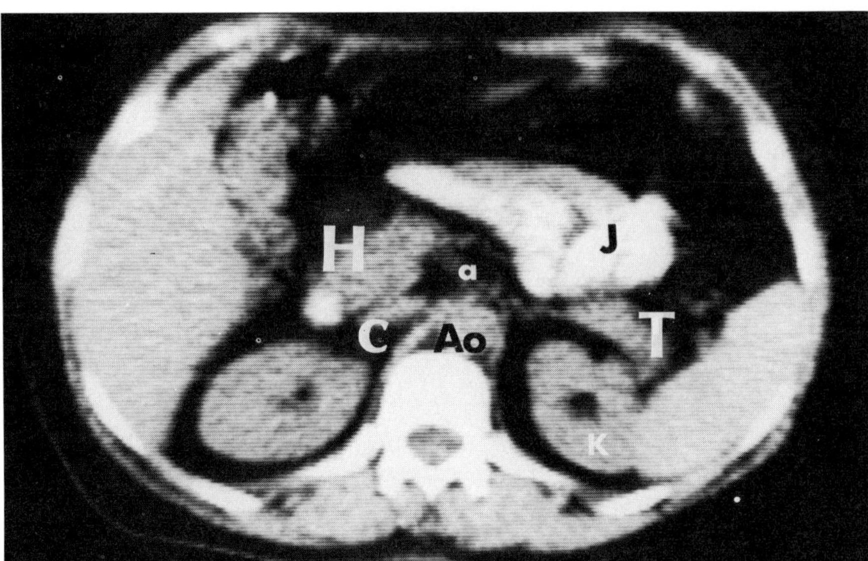

FIGURE 1. The tail (T) of the pancreas lies very close to the hilum of the spleen and arches in front of the left kidney. The head (H) lies in front of the inferior vena cava (C). Note radiopaque contrast material in the jejunum (J). The aorta (Ao) and the superior mesenteric artery (a) are located in the midline.

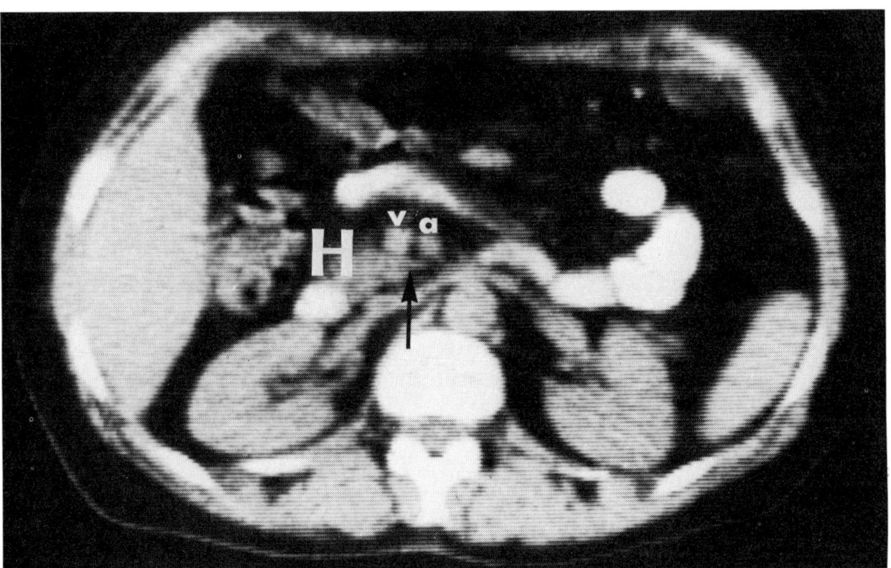

FIGURE 2. The lower portion of the pancreatic head (H) and the uncinate process (arrow) are demonstrated on this more caudad scan. Note the superior mesenteric vein (V) and artery (a) in front of the uncinate process. Both renal arteries are also seen at this level.

of the body of the pancreas and the lateral portion of the head of the pancreas (Figure 3a and b). The location of the distal splenic and portal veins can sometimes be detected by scanning soon after the injection of intravenous contrast material if this proves necessary. The contrast material increases the density of these vessels relative to that of the pancreas. In thin patients, the anterior margin is often just beneath the anterior abdominal wall, while in fatter patients the pancreas is more deeply located. Examination of the slightly obese patient is advantageous because the abdominal fat planes are ample and clearly separate adjacent intra-abdominal organs of similar density.

A relatively standardized technique for the examination of the pancreas by CT is now being used at most institutions. Usually the first scan is obtained at the level of the xyphoid and subsequent scans are obtained at 1.5 cm intervals. Generally, these scans are done in deep inspiration with breath held for the required 20 or 30 seconds. In our experience, greater than 90 percent of all patients are able to suspend respiration for as long as 30 seconds. In order to delineate the unequivocally normal pancreas, approximately 5 to 10 scans are required. A physician is present to review the scans immediately. If the pancreas is clearly abnormal or clearly normal, the examination is generally terminated. However, if the results are equivocal, a repeat examination is conducted, scanning again at 1.5 cm intervals. Oral contrast material is generally given for the second examination, using a 4 percent solution of oral Hypaque®. The patient is then asked to lie on his right side for approximately 5 minutes to ensure filling of the duodenum and distal small bowel (Figures 1–3). One millilitre of spasmolytic agent (glucagon) is injected intramuscularly (occasionally intravenously) and the scans are then repeated with the patient supine. Intravenous contrast material has proved to be of little value in evaluating the normal pancreas. Occasionally, a right side down decubitus scan will prove to be of better value in defining the head of the pancreas.[2]

The pancreas can be oriented horizontally with respect to the long axis of the body or it can be more vertically oriented, or even S-shaped. The number of scans needed to examine the entire pancreas is determined by this orientation. This number can vary from three scans, in the case of the horizontally oriented pancreas, to as many as eight scans in the pancreas that is relatively vertically oriented.

As with other organs of the body, there is some variation in the size of the pancreas. It tends to be relatively larger in young patients and becomes somewhat smaller with advancing age. Evaluation of the size alone does not take into account other factors that must be considered in determining whether a pancreas is normal or abnormal. Guidelines relating the size of the pancreas to the size of the vertebral body are reasonable. However, various anatomical variations should be kept in mind.

Haaga and Alfidi[3] compared the width of the pancreas with the width of the transverse diameter of the vertebral body. This measurement was expressed as a ratio of the pancreatic width over the vertebral body width. The ratio for the widest diameter of the tail and body in 59 patients was 0.5(+ or

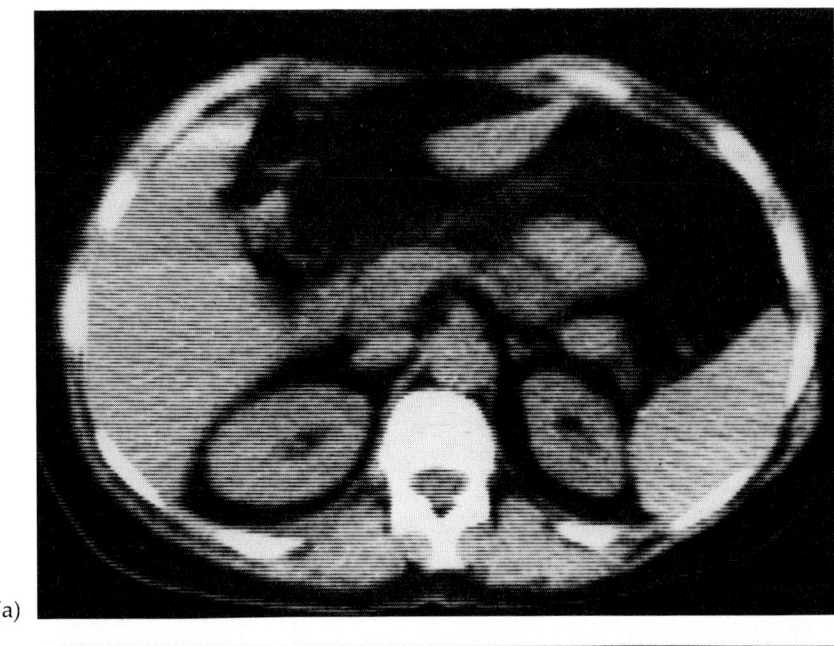

(a)

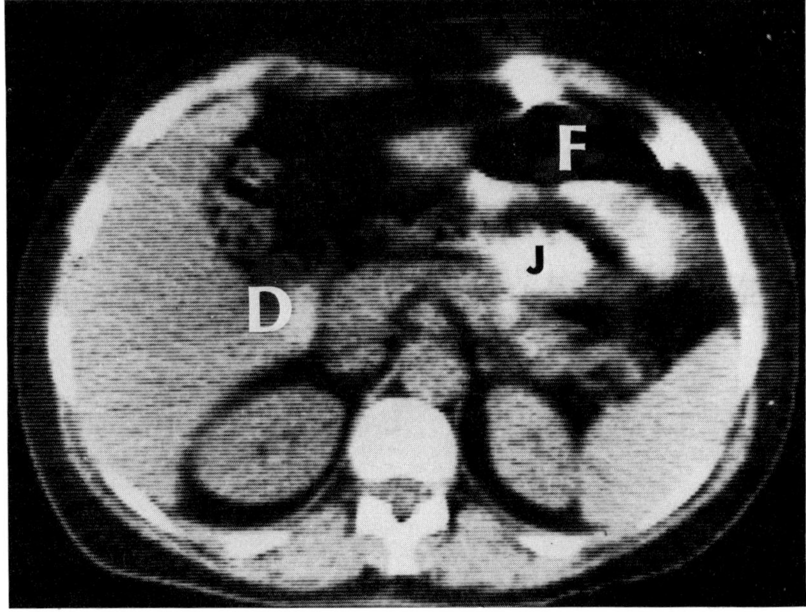

(b)

FIGURE 3. Figure 3a shows a scan through the head, neck and body of the pancreas before oral contrast material has been administered. Figure 3b shows the excellent definition of the gastric fundus (F), second duodenum (D) and jejunum (J) afforded by the contrast material.

− 0.1). The ratio of the head to the vertebral body could be determined in only 52 of the 59 patients. In these 52 the ratio was 0.6(+ or − 0.1). In view of this information, a useful yardstick for evaluating the size of the pancreas is the transverse diameter of the vertebral body. The tail and body should measure at least one third of the widest transverse diameter and yet be no greater than two thirds. The width of the head should be no greater than the full transverse diameter of the vertebral body. This is somewhat greater than the measurement given because, when the patient is examined in the right decubitus position, the pancreas changes its position, making the head somewhat wider.

The organ tends to taper uniformly from head to tail but occasionally the midportion of the body can be thinner than both the head and tail (Figures 1 and 3). Deviations from these two configurations should be viewed with suspicion.

The margins of the pancreas are usually quite distinct, especially in patients with ample retroperitoneal fat. The margins are often smooth, but occasionally a faint lobulation is present. In children and in very thin debilitated patients with little retroperitoneal fat, margins are difficult to see. In addition, the margins can be difficult to see in patients who have had previous surgery that has resulted in the obliteration of the peripancreatic fat plane. Artifacts due to respiratory motion and peristaltic motion also can obscure the margins.

The density of the normal pancreas is uniform from head to tail. In the normal organ there is no calcification or areas of increased or decreased density, and the normal pancreatic duct system cannot be seen. The organ is less dense than liver and approximately equal in density to the spleen, kidneys and skeletal muscle. The injection of intravenous contrast material raises the overall density of the pancreas uniformly.

The normal pancreas without contrast material measures approximately 30–45 H (Hounsfield units), and with intravenous contrast material 60–85 H. Adenocarcinoma and lymphoma are in approximately the same range. Thus, detection of disease depends on recognizing an alteration in the size and/or morphology of the gland. Limitations of CT scanning still exist in evaluating small subclinical lesions.

Diagnostic Ultrasound

With the advent of gray-scale ultrasonography and recent improvements in ultrasound instrumentation and scanning techniques, detailed anatomy of the pancreas is now observed in up to 90 percent of the patient population.[4] With gray-scale instrumentation simple sector scans can be performed, which has allowed accurate identification of vascular landmarks, so important in localizing the pancreas. By avoiding compound scanning, movement is eliminated and the pancreas is separated more easily from adjacent structures. Secondly, gray-scale instrumentation, by recording both specular and back-scattered echoes, permits a display of the tissue consistency of the normal pancreas. This is especially important in detecting pancreatic disease, since pathology may alter not only the size and contour of the organ, but also its ultrasonic tissue consistency.

Anatomy Important in Ultrasonic Localization of the Pancreas

Although normal anatomy has been previously discussed, certain anatomical landmarks bear emphasis in the ultrasonic localization of the pancreas. Its intimate relationship with the abdominal vasculature, particularly the portal venous system, is important.[5] The splenic vein originating in the hilum of the spleen courses to the right, immediately posterior to the body and tail of the pancreas, often forming a groove in the dorsal surface of the organ. Although its course is sometimes variable, it provides the most reliable landmark for the body and tail in transverse section. The splenic vein joins the superior mesenteric vein just to the right of midline to form the portal vein in a groove in the dorsal surface of the pancreas, marking its anatomic neck. The portal vein runs cranially, crossing the inferior vena cava, where it marks the most cephalad border of the pancreatic head. Thus, the head is localized just anterior to the inferior vena cava and caudal to the crossing by the portal vein. The primitive ventral bud which becomes the uncinate process is the only portion of the pancreas that lies dorsal to the portal venous system, often seen extending just posterior to the superior mesenteric vein (Figure 2).

The superior mesenteric artery usually is seen arising from the aorta immediately behind the body of the pancreas and adjacent to the superior mesenteric vein. The left renal vein provides an additional landmark for the body of the pancreas as it is seen coursing transversely from the left kidney to the inferior vena cava, passing between the superior mesenteric artery and the aorta.

The celiac axis arising from the anterior surface of the aorta limits the cephalad extent of the body of the pancreas. Its branches, the splenic and hepatic arteries, are more variable and, although they may become more tortuous with age, provide additional landmarks for the cephalad extent of the tail and head of the pancreas respectively. The gastroduodenal artery, a branch which descends caudally from the hepatic artery, is seen occasionally, accurately marking the anterior surface of the pancreatic head. The common bile duct, located anteriorly and to the left of the portal vein in the hepatogastric ligament, is sometimes seen coursing caudally on the posterior surface of the pancreas before entering the ampulla of Vater, providing accurate localization.

The gallbladder is anterior to the head of the pancreas and usually to the right, though it occasionally may lie immediately anterior to the head, providing an ideal acoustic window. Gas in the duodenum may provide accurate localization of the lateral aspect of the pancreatic head, though occasionally gas in the duodenal bulb produces acoustic shadowing, obscuring detail.

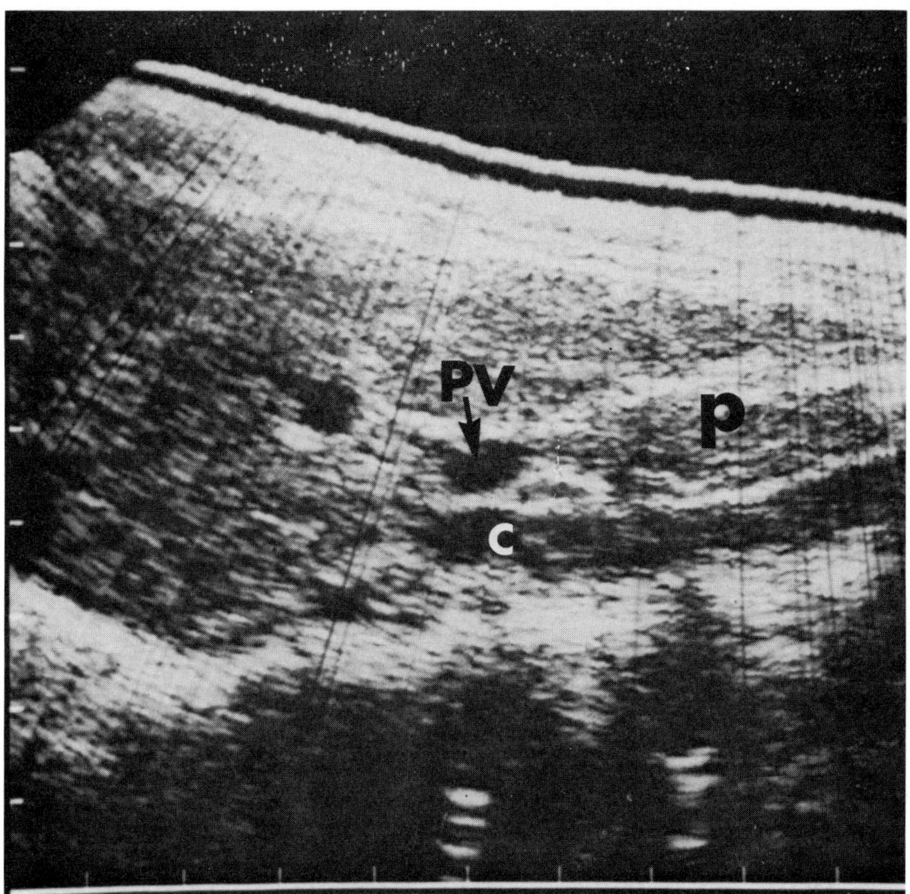

FIGURE 4. A right parasagittal scan over the inferior vena cava (C) localizes the head of the pancreas (P) just anterior to it and immediately caudal to the crossing of the portal vein (PV).

Technique

Ultrasound examination is performed on the patient in a fasting state and early in the morning so as to avoid intestinal gas from swallowed air. Cigarette smoking also leads to swallowed air, and patients are asked to abstain prior to the examination. We have not found that administration of Simethicone or other "degassing agents" has been helpful. Using a commercially available gray-scale B-scanner in the average size patient a 2.25 MHz transducer focused at about 7 cm will give the best images. In thin patients or in children, a 3.5 MHz transducer focused at about 5 cm will give superior images. In obese patients, a 2.25 MHz transducer with a longer focus of 9 – 10 cm may be necessary, and occasionally one may have to resort to using a 1.6 MHz transducer to obtain adequate penetration. The patient is initially ex-

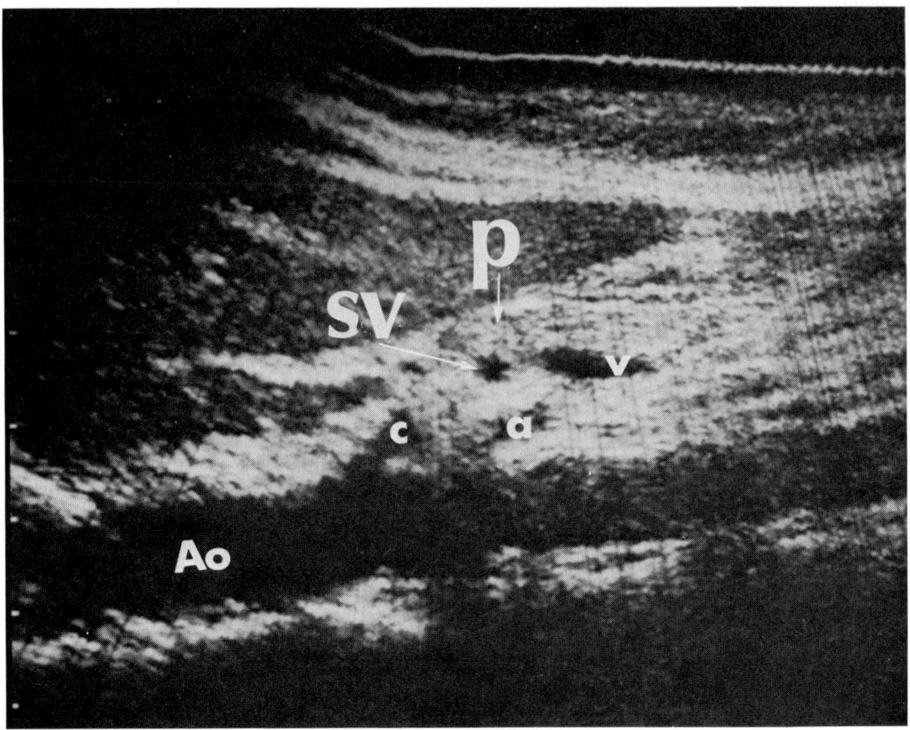

FIGURE 5. A midline sagittal scan defines the superior mesenteric vein (V), splenic vein (SV), aorta (Ao), superior mesenteric artery (a) and celiac artery (C). The pancreas (P) is located anterior to the splenic vein and superior mesenteric vein.

amined in the supine position, and a generous amount of mineral oil is applied to the abdomen as a coupling agent. Scans are carried out in suspended inspiration to arrest respiratory motion and to provide an acoustic window through the descended liver. Additionally, full inspiration dilates the portal venous system, facilitating its identification.

Since the pancreas is a transversely oriented organ which moves in a craniocaudad direction with respiration, the quickest and most reliable means of localizing the pancreas is to begin by performing parasagittal scans. First, a right parasagittal scan over the inferior vena cava localizes the head of the pancreas just anterior to it and immediately caudal to the crossing by the portal vein (Figure 4). Serial sagittal scans are then performed over the midline localizing the superior mesenteric vein and, slightly to the left, the superior mesenteric artery seen arising from the anterior surface of the aorta (Figure 5). The pancreas is identified in the angle formed by the left lobe of the liver and the superior mesenteric vessels. Often the hepatic and splenic arteries are seen in cross section which provides a landmark for the cephalad extent of the pancreas. A circular or donut-shaped density representing the antrum of the stomach is often seen just caudal and anterior to the pancreatic tissue,

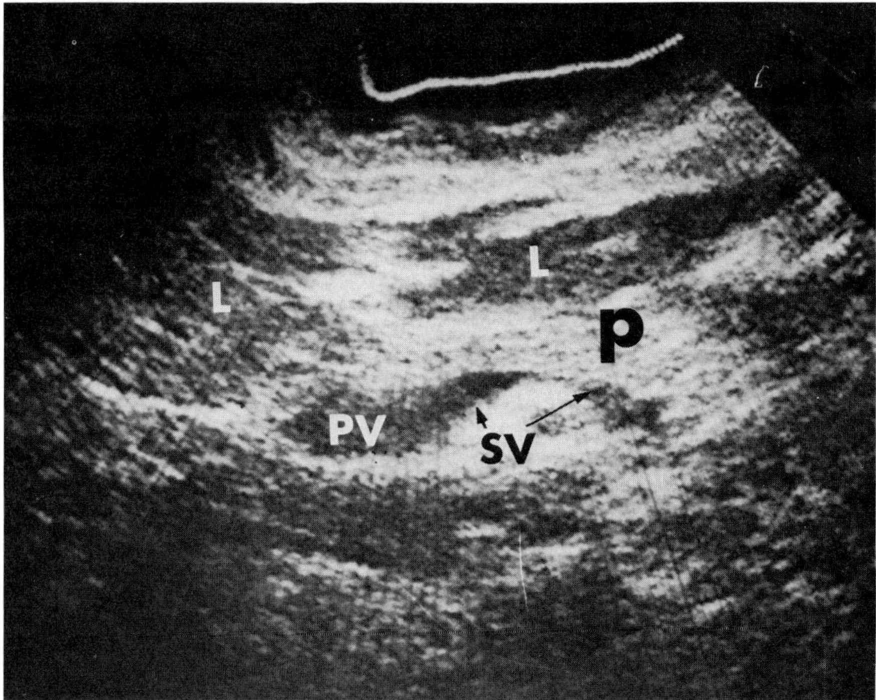

FIGURE 6. A transverse scan defines the splenic vein (SV) posterior to the body and tail of the pancreas (P). On the right, its junction with the superior mesenteric vein to form the portal vein (PV) posterior to the neck of the pancreas is seen. Note the difference in echogenicity between the liver (L) and pancreas.

and should not be confused with it. This may be easily confirmed by asking the patient to drink water, filling the antrum with fluid. In parasagittal section, the splenic vein is often seen just posterior to the body and tail of the pancreas (Figure 5) and with serial parasagittal sections its axis can be quickly determined, thus generally establishing the axis of the body and tail of the pancreas.

Next, scans are carried out transversely, following the axis of the pancreas determined from the parasagittal scans. First, the splenic vein is easily identifiable posterior to the body and tail of the pancreas, and it can be traced to the right to its union with the superior mesenteric vein where it forms the portal vein posterior to the neck of the pancreas (Figure 6). The superior mesenteric artery in cross section and the long axis of the left renal vein coursing between it and the aorta provide additional vascular landmarks for the body of the pancreas. Often, a single scan will include (from right to left) the lumen of the gallbladder, gas in the duodenum, the head, body, and tail of the pancreas lying just anterior to the upper pole of the left kidney.

In cases where intestinal gas compromises visualization of the normal pan-

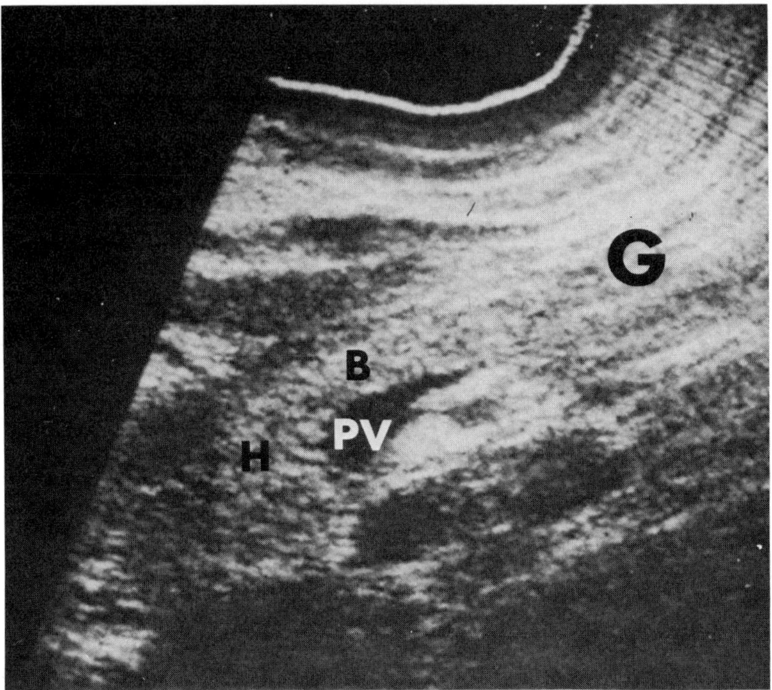

FIGURE 7. (a) A transverse scan clearly demonstrates the pancreatic head (H) and body (B), splenic vein and portal vein (PV). On the left, overlying bowel gas (G) obscures the pancreatic tail.

creas, manual pressure is usually sufficient to displace it. Occasionally, placing the patient in a slight left lateral decubitus position will shift the liver and displace duodenal and gastric antral gas which obscures the head of the pancreas. In more difficult cases, we have found that filling the stomach with fluid may markedly improve the technical quality of the examination. The patient is asked to drink as much fluid as possible (usually 500cc is sufficient) while in the left lateral decubitus position to retain fluid in the gastric fundus.

Scanning is then begun in the supine position several minutes after the microbubbles have dispersed. Transverse scans (Figure 7a and b) demonstrate the tail of the pancreas behind the fluid-filled stomach. A more recent technique described at this center[6] involves positioning the patient in the right decubitus position, thus filling the gastric antrum, and following the water bolus into the duodenum outlining the pancreatic head.

Finally, the patient is placed in the prone position and transverse and sagittal scans are performed through the left renal bed, revealing the pancreatic tail sandwiched between the fluid-filled gastric fundus and the left kidney.

Variations in normal size of the pancreas have been reported.[5, 7-9] We feel

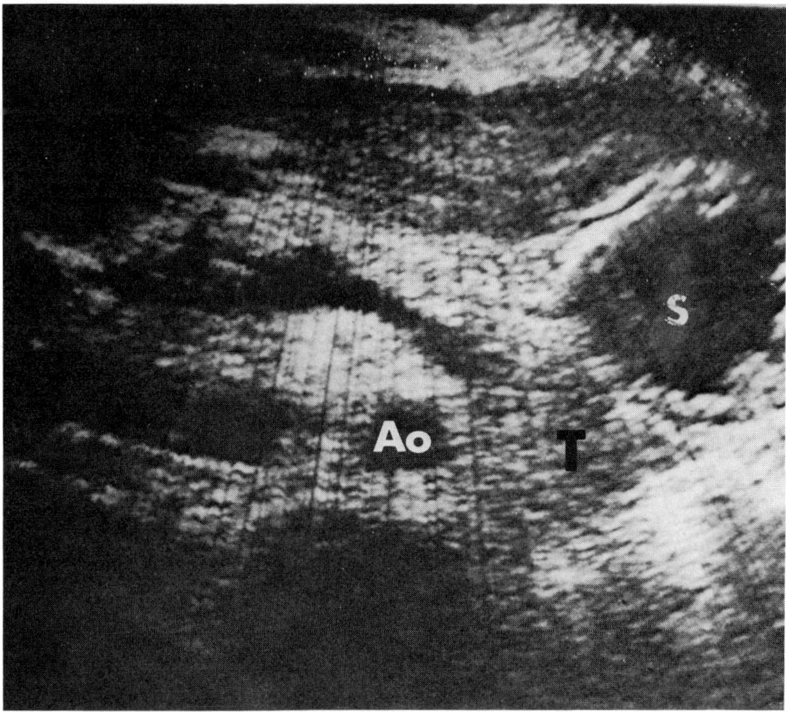

(b) The stomach (S), now filled with water, can be used as an acoustic window to clearly visualize the tail (T). The aorta (Ao) is seen.

that in a good technical examination with identification of the vascular landmarks, a maximum AP dimension of the head of 2.5 cm will encompass 95 percent of normal patients.[4] The upper limits of normal AP dimension should be no larger than 1.5 cm and 2.0 cm for the neck and body of the pancreas. Less accurate data are available for the size of the tail, but its dimensions should be no larger than those of the pancreatic head. The normal pancreas appears slightly thicker in young patients and decreases in size with advancing age.[7]

With gray-scale instrumentation, an ultrasonic "tissue consistency" is recorded and should be evaluated in addition to size and contour. In most patients a definite echo consistency is observed which produces higher-level back-scattered echoes than the normal liver. This is best observed in transverse section by comparing the left lobe of the liver with the pancreas and slowly decreasing the overall gain until the liver echoes are seen to "drop out" while the internal echoes of the normal pancreas are maintained (Figures 6 and 7). Occasionally in examinations which are technically poor owing to obesity or intestinal gas, the tissue consistency of the gland cannot be separated from that of surrounding tissues. In these cases, however, use of the vascular landmarks permits accurate localization of the space the pancreas occupies and its size can be determined.

With a good knowledge of anatomy and adherence to technical criteria, an accurate appraisal can usually be made of the size, contour and ultrasonic consistency of the normal pancreas, providing a basis for the early detection of pancreatic disease.

References

1. Sheedy PF, Stephens DH, Hattery RR, MacCarthy RL and Williamson B: Computed tomography of the pancreas. Radiol Clin N Amer 15:349–366, 1977.
2. Haaga JR and Alfidi RJ: Computed tomographic scanning of the pancreas. Radiol Clin N Amer 15:367–376, 1977.
3. Haaga JR, Alfidi RJ, Zelch MG, Meany TE, Boller M, Gonzalez L and Jelden GL: Computed tomography of the pancreas. Radiol 120:589–595, 1976.
4. de Graaff CS, Taylor KJW, Simonds BD and Rosenfield AT: Gray-scale echography of the pancreas: re-evaluation of normal size. Radiol (In press).
5. Doust BD and Pearce JD: Gray-scale ultrasonic properties of the normal and inflamed pancreas. Radiol 120:653–657, 1976.
6. Crade M, Taylor KJW, Rosenfield AT: Water distention of the gut in the evaluation of pancreas by ultrasound. Amer J Roentgenol 131:227–230, 1978.
7. Weill F, Schraub A, Eisenscher A, and Bourgoin A: Ultrasonography of the normal pancreas—success rate and criteria for normality. Radiol 123:417–423, 1977.
8. Simonds BD: In Atlas of Gray Scale Ultrasonography, ed. Taylor KJW, P. 132. Edinburgh: Churchill Livingstone, 1977.
9. Haber K, Freimanis AK, Asher WM: Demonstration and dimensional analysis of the normal pancreas with gray-scale echography. Amer J Roentgenol 126:624–628, 1976.

Diagnosis of Pancreatic Disease by Ultrasound and Computed Tomography

W. F. SAMPLE
D. A. SARTI

Before ultrasound and, more recently, computed body tomography were developed, pancreatic abnormalities were noninvasively imaged by indirect means. Plain films of the abdomen might show suspicious gas patterns in acute pancreatitis, extraluminal air in pancreatic abscesses, and calcifications in chronic pancreatitis and some tumors. Pancreatic enlargements were detectable by their indirect displacement of the gastrointestinal tract, usually demonstrated after the administration of oral contrast agents. Functional defects indicating tumor or inflammation could be detected with selenomethionine scintigraphy. However, similar changes secondary to dietary factors and other nonpancreatic diseases were frequently encountered, leading to a significant false positive rate. More invasive techniques such as angiography, endoscopic retrograde cannulation of the pancreatic ducts (ERCP) and percutaneous transhepatic cholangiography have improved the detection accuracy of pancreatic disease but are associated with some morbidity and therefore are not ideal screening procedures.

Ultrasound and computed tomography are both capable of directly and noninvasively imaging the pancreas.[1-6] Each modality utilizes a different form of energy and monitors different tissue characteristics. These basic factors impose certain strengths and limitations which are fortunately offsetting. A considerable experience with both modalities in the diagnosis of pancreatic disease has now been reported and serves as the basis for this review.

General Considerations

The images generated by computed tomography are based on differences in the linear attenuation of X-rays which, in turn, are related to the density and anatomic number of tissues. No biological tissues completely attenuate the 120 – 140 keV energies and, therefore, all parts of the body can be examined. The accumulation of data for the reconstructive process requires time. Although scanners capable of obtaining the necessary data in one second are now available, the majority of the data involving the pancreas have been generated with 18-second scanners. As a result, biological motion artifacts have to be considered and represent one important limitation in the pancreatic area.

With 18-second scanners, respiration can be voluntarily suspended in 80 – 90 percent of patients. However, peristalsis must also be reduced with intravenous antispasmodics to obtain high quality images.[7]

In spite of the spatial and contrast resolution possible with 18-second computed tomographic scanners, the intra-abdominal organs are not distinguishable unless they are separated by retroperitoneal fat. Furthermore, oral iodinated contrast agents must be utilized to identify accurately the various portions of the gastrointestinal tract surrounding the pancreas.[2, 7-12]

With the limitations of an 18-second scanner, optimal computed tomograms of the pancreas are obtained in patients with a medium to obese body habitus. In addition, patients must be capable of suspending respiration for the length of the scan, have no contraindication to the use of antispasmodics and be able to tolerate oral iodinated contrast agents. Preliminary studies indicate that in 80 – 90 percent of patients these requirements are met and diagnostic computed tomograms of the pancreas can be achieved.[2, 7, 8, 10, 12-14] In addition, it has been noted that the body and tail of the pancreas are more often optimally evaluated than the head.[9, 15]

The total reconstruction time for computed tomograms obtained with an 18-second scanner has been relatively long. Examinations of the pancreas may take from 30 to 60 minutes. As a result, patient throughput is slow and the cost is high. These economic considerations are important determinants in the selection of a screening procedure for pancreatic disease.

With ultrasound, the reflection, scatter and attenuation of sound energy by biological tissues, based on elasticity and density, are imaged. The natural contrast between the various abdominal organs is excellent and most organs can be identified by means of their specific internal graytone texture as well as their position.[1, 3-6, 9, 16-19]

High frequency soundwaves do not penetrate all biological tissues. Sound is rapidly attenuated by bone, totally reflected by air and severely scattered by subcutaneous fat. One or all of these biological tissues may be encountered when trying to image all of the pancreas. As a result, the optimal patient for ultrasonic examination has a medium to thin body habitus and a collapsed or fluid-filled gastrointestinal tract. Existing reports indicate that diagnostic studies of the pancreas are obtained in 80–90 percent of patients and that the head and body regions are more frequently visualized than the tail.[1, 3, 5, 6, 20]

Limited high resolution ultrasonograms can be obtained in one second. As a result, biological motion is not a significant problem. In addition, a complete examination of the pancreas from a variety of anatomic approaches can be obtained in 15 to 30 minutes. Patient throughput is therefore good and the financial considerations are favorable for a screening procedure. Finally, the lack of demonstrable toxicity to the sound intensities generated by existing equipment makes the examination applicable to all ages and during pregnancy.[21]

General Criteria for Pancreatic Disease

The direct signs of an abnormal pancreas include focal or generalized enlargement and changes in texture (Figures 1–14). Ultrasonic studies designed to determine the upper limits of normal for the anterior–posterior diameter of the various regions of the pancreas have suggested: 2.5–3.5 cm for the head; 1.5–3.0 cm for the body; and 2.8–3.5 cm for the tail.[1, 5, 6, 20] A similar study with computed tomography indicated anterior–posterior diameters of 3.0 cm for the head, 2.5 cm for the body and 2.0 cm for the tail.[2] However, three normal variants of the size relationships of the head, body and tail of the pancreas have been described: sausage-shaped, dumbbell-shaped and a gradual tapering.[2] As a result, biological variations always make measurements subject to error.

A recognizable change in texture is a more reliable direct sign of early pancreatic disease. On ultrasonograms, solid areas of decreased echogenicity are observed with edema, neoplastic infiltration and some types of scarring (Figures 1, 3, 11 and 13).[4, 9, 14, 16, 18, 19, 22] Areas of increased echogenicity are observed with fibrofatty infiltration, calcification, mucin production and air (Figures 5 and 7).[14, 17-20, 22, 23] Fluid regions can be seen with cysts, pseudocysts, liquefied hemorrhage, abscesses and marked edema (Figure 9).[14, 16, 18, 19, 22-27]

On computed tomograms, a slight decrease in the linear attenuation of X-rays may be seen with edema, neoplastic infiltration, fibrofatty infiltration and mucin production (Figures 2 and 8).[8, 10-12, 14, 15, 20, 28-31] An even lower attenuation value is observed in fluid areas secondary to abscess, pseudocyst and liquefied hemorrhage (Figure 10). The lowest linear attenuation values are seen in air-containing abscesses. Increased areas of linear attenuation are associated with calcifications and occasionally fresh hemorrhage (Figure 6).

Indirect signs of pancreatic disease are dilatation of the pancreatic and/or biliary ducts (Figures 15 and 16).[8-10, 12, 29, 32] Ultrasound and computed tomography have both been shown to be highly accurate in the detection of biliary dilation. Similarly, a dilated pancreatic duct can be resolved by either modality (Figures 15 and 16). However, care must be taken not to mistake the an-

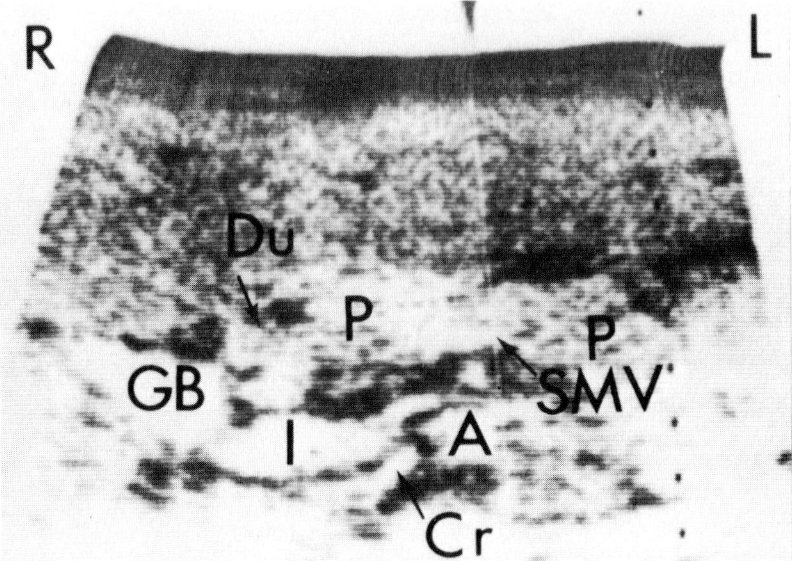

FIGURE 1. Transverse gray-scale sonogram through the head and body region of the pancreas (P), demonstrating a solid type of decreased echogenicity in the head region without definite enlargment. Clinical and laboratory findings confirmed the diagnosis of acute pancreatitis. (Du = duodenum; GB = gallbladder; I = inferior vena cava; A = aorta; Cr = crus of the diaphragm; SMV = superior mesenteric vein).

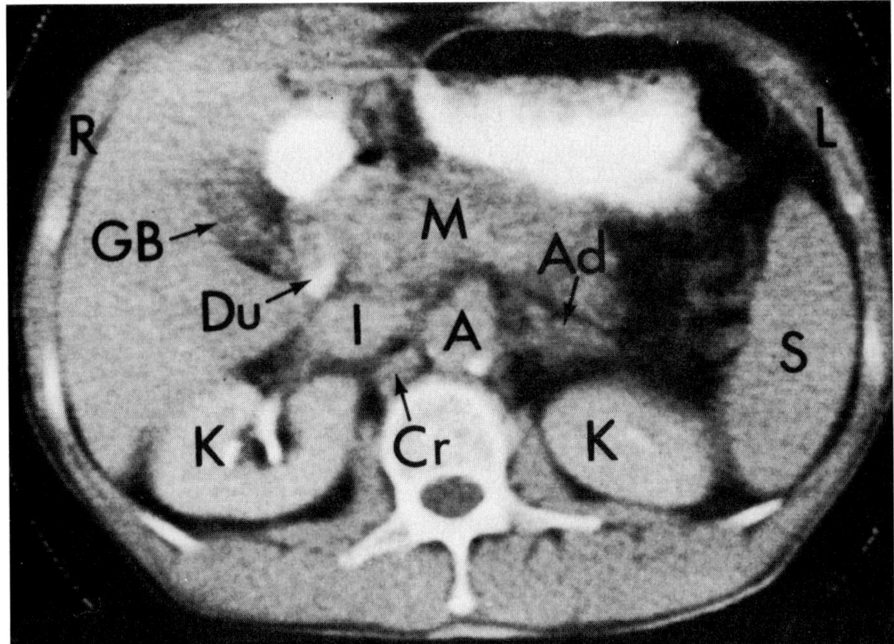

FIGURE 2. Transverse computed tomogram through the head and body region of the pancreas, showing a mass type enlargement (M) with a slightly decreased patchy attenuation. Clinical and laboratory findings confirmed the diagnosis of acute pancreatitis. (GB = gallbladder; Du = duodenum; K = kidneys; I = inferior vena cava; A = aorta; Cr = crus of the diaphragm; Ad = left adrenal; S = spleen).

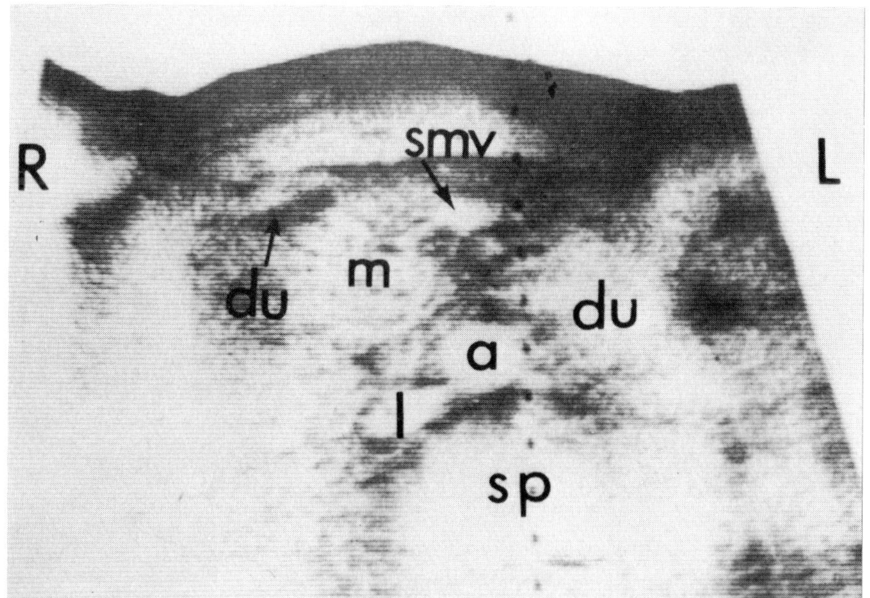

FIGURE 3. Transverse gray-scale sonogram showing a mass type enlargement (M) of the head of the pancreas, with an abnormal decreased solid type echogenicity. A diagnosis of chronic pancreatitis was established at surgery. (du = duodenum; smv = superior mesenteric vein; I = inferior vena cava; a = aorta; sp = spine).

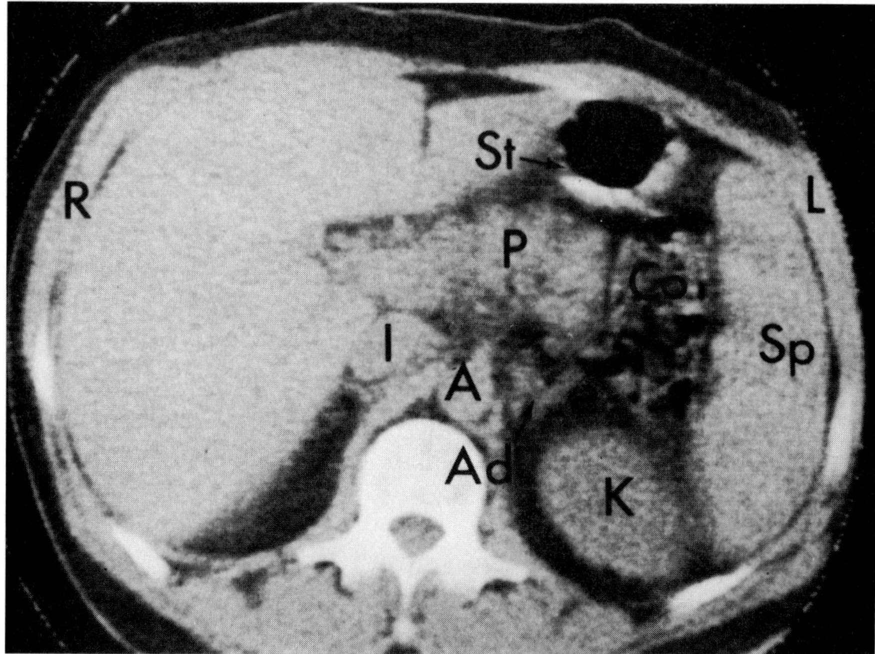

FIGURE 4. Transverse computed tomogram through the body of the pancreas (P), showing enlargement but without abnormal attenuation value. Biopsies at surgery demonstrated chronic pancreatitis. (St = stomach; I = inferior vena cava; A = aorta; Ad = left adrenal; K = left kidney; Co = colon; Sp = spleen).

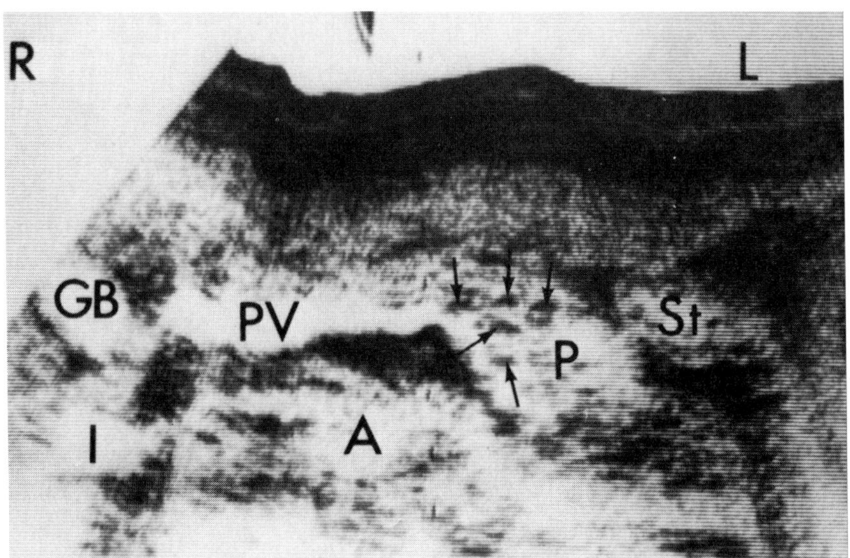

FIGURE 5. Transverse gray-scale sonogram through the body—tail region of the pancreas (P), demonstrating punctate areas of increased echogenicity (arrows) compatible with calcifications. Biopsies at surgery confirmed the diagnosis of chronic pancreatitis.
(GB = gallbladder; I = inferior vena cava; A = aorta; PV = portal vein; St = stomach).

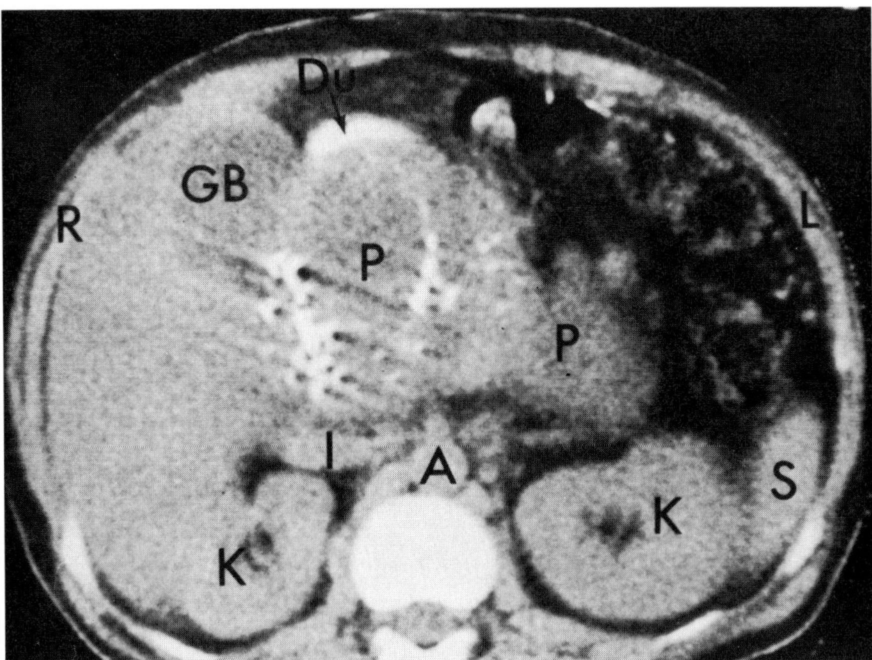

FIGURE 6. Transverse computed tomogram showing an enlargement of the head and body of the pancreas (P) containing multiple high-density areas consistent with calcification. Biopsies at surgery confirmed chronic pancreatitis. (GB = gallbladder; Du = duodenum; I = inferior vena cava; A = aorta; K = kidney; S = spleen).

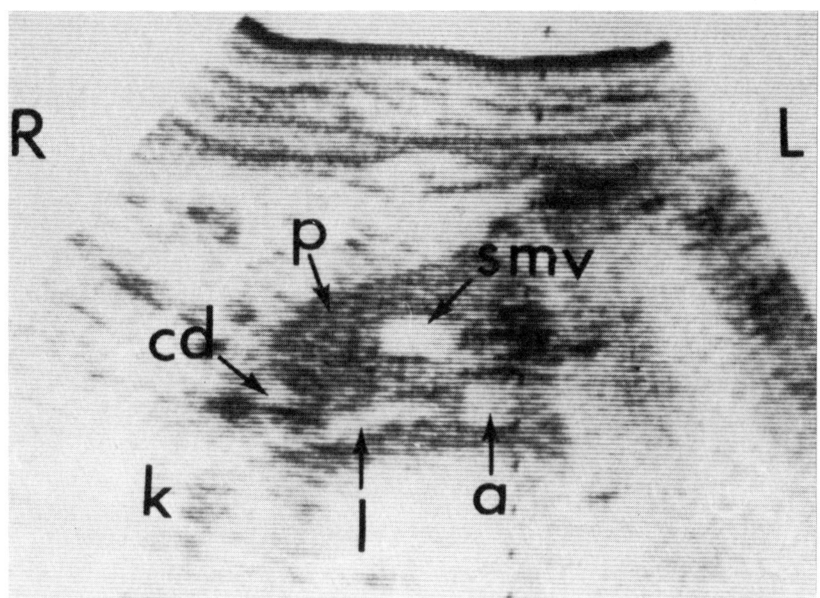

FIGURE 7. Transverse gray-scale sonogram through the head of the pancreas (p) which shows a high level of echogenicity when compared to the adjacent liver. This form of chronic pancreatitis may be difficult to distinguish from normal pancreas. (cd = common duct; k = kidney; a = aorta; i = inferior vena cava; smv = superior mesenteric vein).

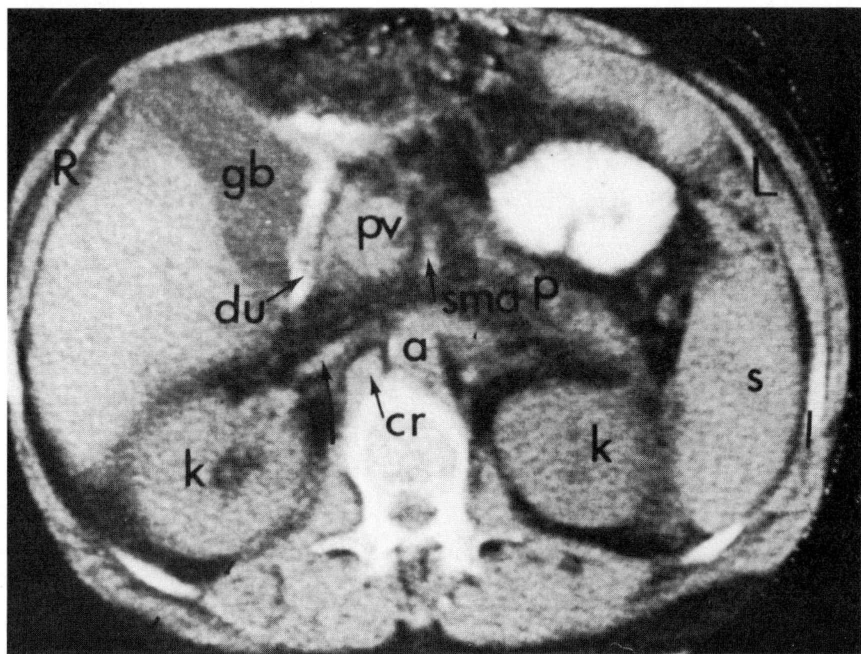

FIGURE 8. Transverse computed tomogram through the pancreas (p), showing a generalized but patchy low attenuation value. These changes may accompany some types of chronic pancreatitis and can be difficult to distinguish from the normal fibro-fatty atrophy of the pancreas that occurs with age. (gb = gallbladder; du = duodenum; pv = portal vein; sma = superior mesenteric artery; a = aorta; I = inferior vena cava; cr = crus of the diaphragm; k = kidney; s = spleen).

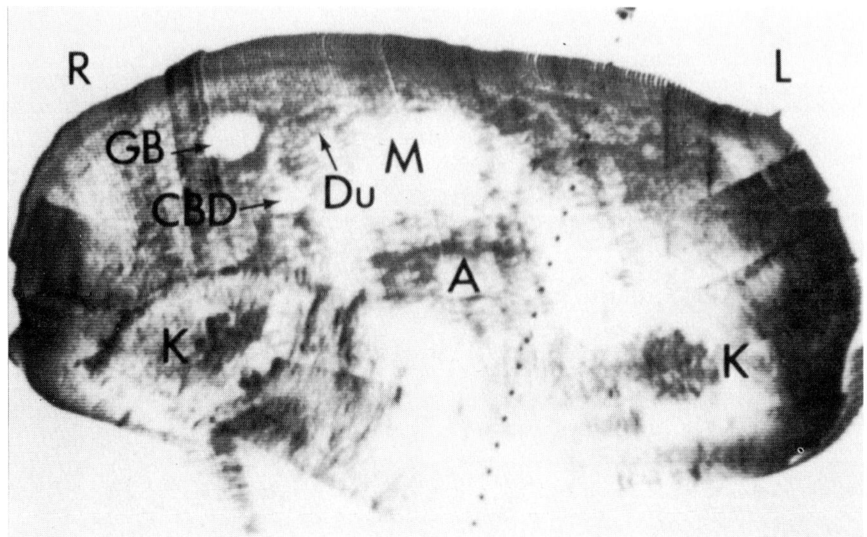

FIGURE 9. Transverse gray-scale sonogram through the head of the pancreas, showing a cystic mass (M) with an irregular wall compatible with a pseudocyst. (GB = gallbladder; CBD = common bile duct; Du = duodenum; A = aorta; K = kidney).

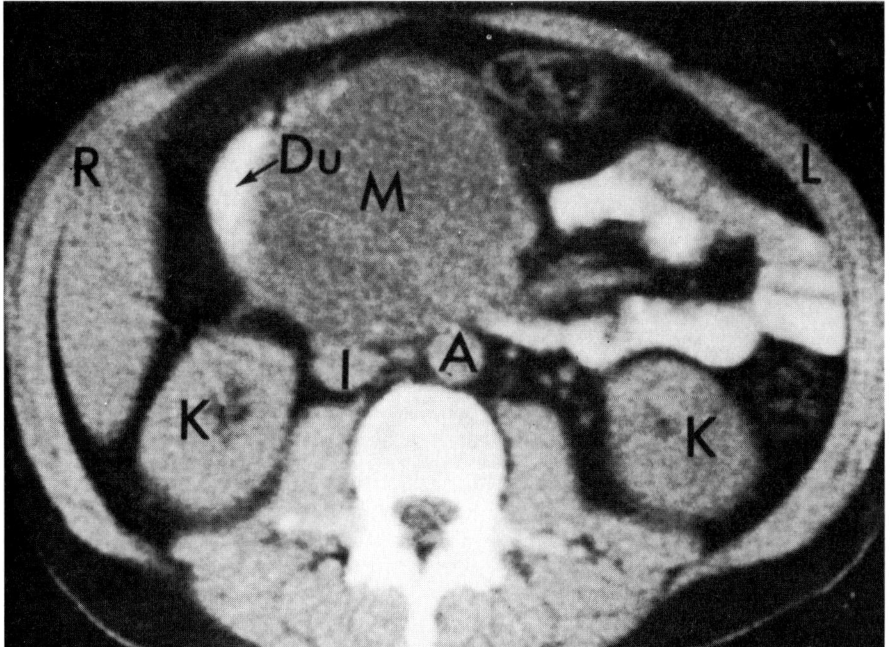

FIGURE 10. Transverse computed tomogram through the head of the pancreas, demonstrating a mass type enlargement (M) with an attenuation value equal to that of water. A pseudocyst was drained at surgery. (Du = duodenum; I = inferior vena cava; A = aorta; K = kidney).

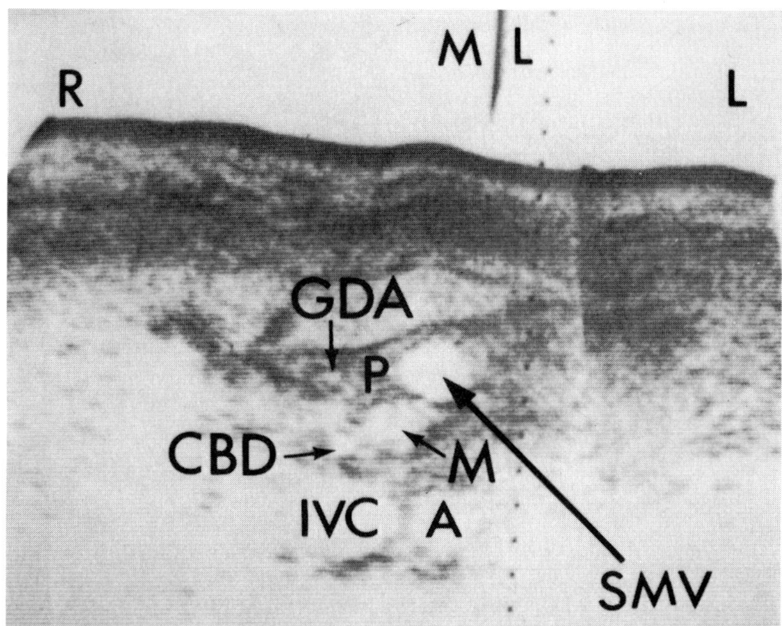

FIGURE 11. Transverse gray-scale sonogram through the head of the pancreas (P), showing a small mass (M) in the region of the uncinate process. The clinical findings were consistent with an insulinoma which was subsequently removed at surgery. (GDA = gastroduodenal artery; CBD = common bile duct; IVC = inferior vena cava; A = aorta; SMV = superior mesenteric vein).

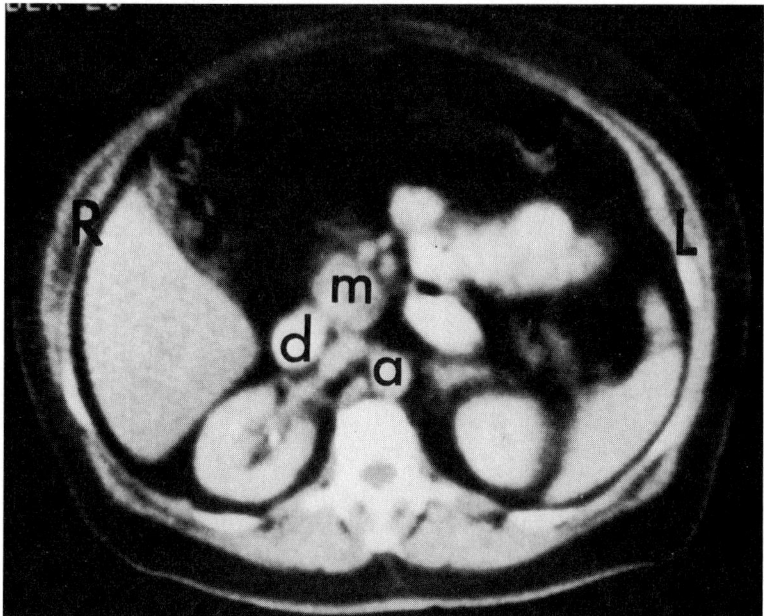

FIGURE 12. Transverse computed tomogram through the head of the pancreas, showing a mass (m) indicated by a rounding of the uncinate process. Clinical findings were consistent with an insulinoma which was subsequently removed at surgery. (d = duodenum; a = aorta).

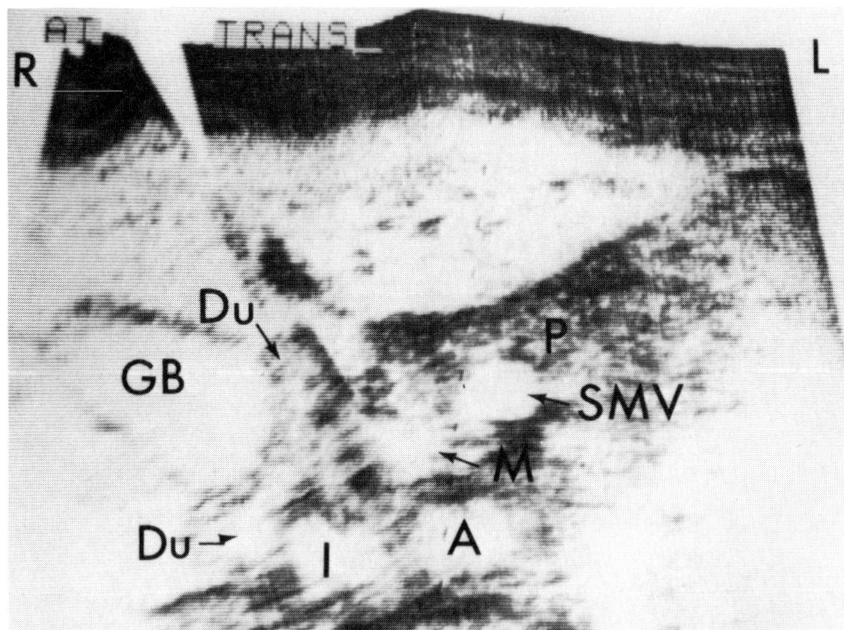

FIGURE 13. Transverse gray-scale sonogram through the head of the pancreas, showing a solid area of abnormal texture (M) which at surgery proved to be a small carcinoma. (GB = gallbladder; Du = duodenum; I = inferior vena cava; A = aorta; SMV = superior mesenteric vein; P = body of pancreas).

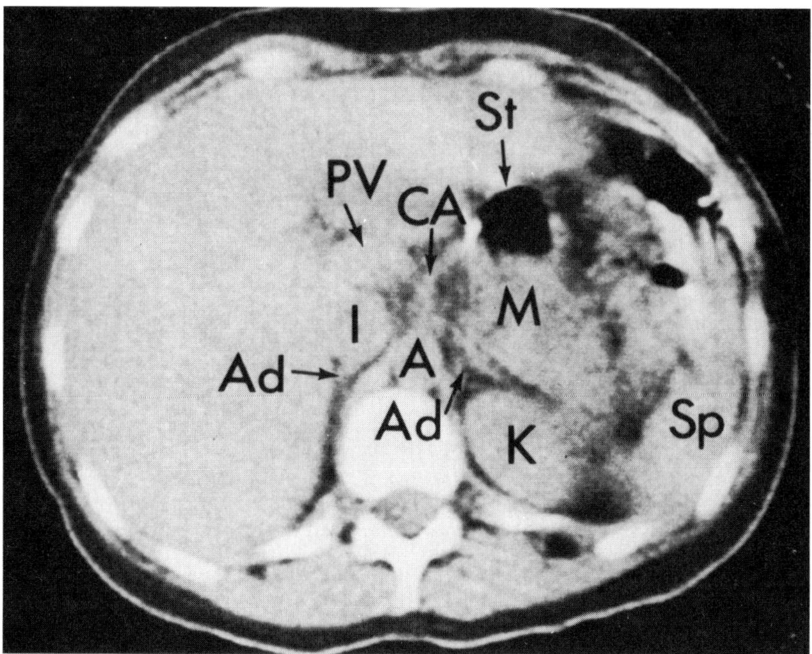

FIGURE 14. Transverse computed tomogram through the body of the pancreas, showing a slight mass type enlargement (M) without an abnormal attenuation value. At surgery, a carcinoma was confirmed. (PV = portal vein; I = inferior vena cava; Ad = adrenal gland; A = aorta; K = left kidney; CA = celiac artery; St = stomach; Sp = spleen).

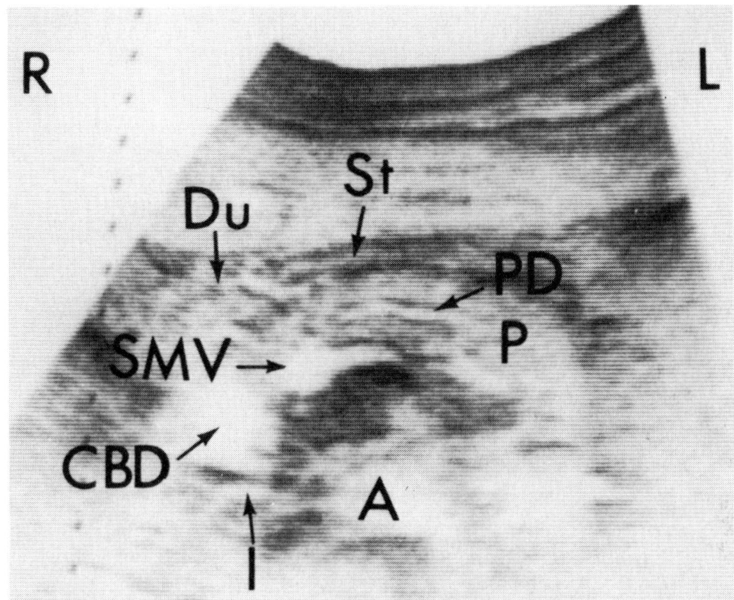

FIGURE 15. Transverse gray-scale sonogram through the pancreas, showing a dilated pancreatic duct (PD) and a dilated common bile duct (CBD). At surgery, a small obstructing pancreatic carcinoma was resected. (Du = duodenum; St = stomach; SMV = superior mesenteric vein; I = inferior vena cava; A = aorta).

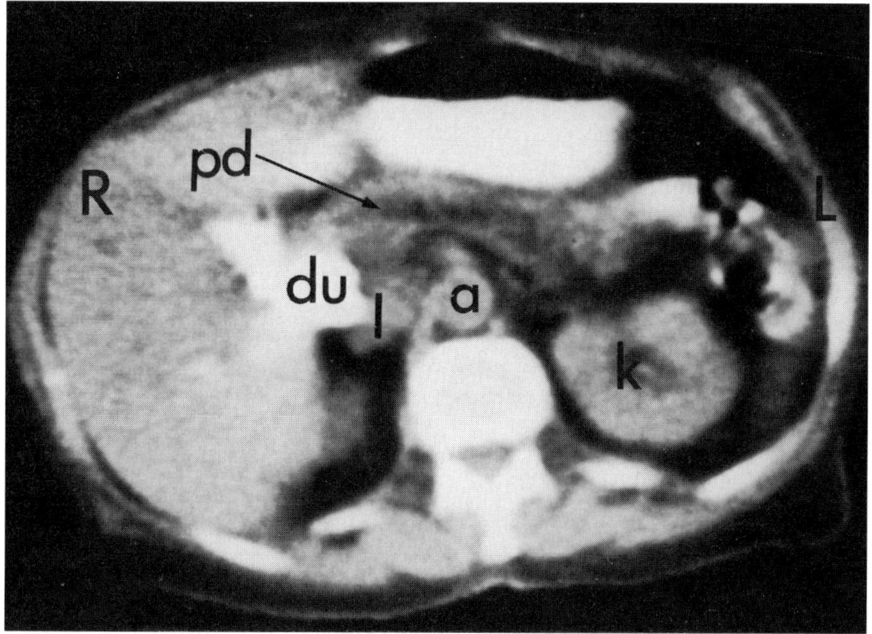

FIGURE 16. Transverse computed tomogram through the pancreas, showing a dilated pancreatic duct (pd). At surgery, a small obstructing carcinoma was removed. (du = duodenum; I = inferior vena cava; a = aorta; k = left kidney).

trum of the stomach on ultrasound and the fat plane between the splenic vein and the pancreas on computed tomograms for a dilated pancreatic duct.[9, 32, 33]

Diagnostic Accuracy

A number of studies determining the accuracy of ultrasound and computed tomography in the diagnosis of pancreatic disease have been reported. Those studies utilizing contemporary instrumentation (gray-scale ultrasound and 18-second or faster computed tomographic scanners) and amenable to decision matrix analysis are summarized in Tables 1 and 2. Although the range of nosological probabilities has been similar, a number of observations not evident in the Tables should be noted.

The diagnosis of pancreatic abnormalities of the tail has been more difficult with ultrasound than with computed tomography.[17, 20] Lesions involving the body of the pancreas have been detected with equal accuracy by both modalities. Diseases of the head of the pancreas have been more accurately detected by ultrasound, although both modalities are accurate in the region of the uncinate process.[15]

Small abnormalities have been detectable with both modalities when they obstruct the biliary or pancreatic ductal systems. However, nonobstructing solid abnormalities of the pancreas frequently do not alter the attenuation of X-rays, whereas they usually alter the acoustical texture. As a result, small, centrally located solid lesions which do not obstruct the ductal systems and do not alter the contour of the pancreas, are more likely to be detected with ultrasound.

Differential Diagnostic Capabilities

Ultrasound and computed tomography are equally effective in differentiating solid from cystic lesions of the pancreas.[12, 14, 16, 20, 24, 29, 30] The attenuation values approach those of water on computed tomograms and the classic findings of fluid are observed on ultrasonograms. Fluid areas are most commonly found with pseudocyst formation associated with acute or chronic relapsing pancreatitis. Additional findings, such as generalized enlargement of the pancreas and calcification, may aid in the differential diagnosis. Small pseudocysts in the tail of the pancreas are frequently better visualized with CT, especially after the administration of intravenous contrast agents. Both ultrasound and CT have been effective in following the course of pseudocysts and demonstrating their maturation or spontaneous dissolution in response to therapy.[25, 26]

However, fluid areas can be associated with abscess formation and some tumors, especially cyst adenomas and cyst adenocarcinomas.[23, 27] In addition, pseudocysts may be complex in nature with loculations, hemorrhage or extensive debris. All of these entities have overlapping attenuation values on

TABLE 1. Accuracy of gray-scale ultrasonography of the pancreas

			Nosological probabilities (%)				
Authors	**No. Cases**	**% Non-diagnostic**	**Sensitivity**	**Specificity**	**False negative**	**False positive**	**Accuracy**
Feinberg et al[35]	32	3	96	100	4	0	97
Ponette et al[14]	45	18	77	93	23	7	84
Lawson[17]	236	15	82	93	18	7	87
Kazam et al[20]	100	15	68	92	32	8	85
Barkin et al[34]	46	2	94	100	6	0	96
Levitt et al[30]	71	20	87	71	13	29	77

TABLE 2. Accuracy of computed tomography of the pancreas

			Nosological probabilities (%)				
Authors	**No. Cases**	**% Non-diagnostic**	**Sensitivity**	**Specificity**	**False negative**	**False positive**	**Accuracy**
Haaga et al[29]	63	—	80	92	20	8	83
Ponette et al[14]	45	20	80	100	20	0	89
Stanley et al[12]	352	8	95	94	5	6	94
Di Magno et al[13]	70	7	84	84	16	16	84
Sheedy et al[10]	90	0	89	87	11	13	88
Kazam et al[20]	100	—	87	92	13	8	90
Ferrucci et al[15]	91	—	77	61	23	39	74

computed tomograms and similar acoustical textures on ultrasound. The presence of air within a fluid mass will usually indicate an abscess. This finding is more specifically identified with computed tomography. Air within a mass may lead to a nondiagnostic ultrasound study or give an echogenic focus that cannot be differentiated from calcification. In some cases, the information from each modality will allow a more specific differential diagnosis.[23] Neither computed tomography nor ultrasound has been reliable in the differentiation of benign and malignant solid masses.[8, 10, 12, 15, 17, 18, 20, 28-31] On computed tomograms, the range of attenuation values observed in acute pancreatitis, chronic pancreatitis and pancreatic neoplasms is similar. In addition, differential enhancement of attenuation values following the administration of intravenous iodinated contrast has not been reliably observed. In many patients, the attenuation values for solid abnormalities are the same as for normal pancreas, and a pathological state is diagnosed only on the basis of localized or diffuse enlargement.

Although most solid abnormalities alter the normal acoustical texture of the pancreas on ultrasonograms, patterns specific for benign or malignant disease have not been found. In general, the echogenicity of solid pancreatic abnormalities is less than that of normal pancreas, which, in turn, is equal to or slightly greater than that of the liver.

If calcifications are discovered with either modality, a benign process is favored. However, some pancreatic tumors may contain calcifications. Furthermore, pancreatic neoplasms occur with a higher incidence in patients with chronic pancreatitis. Therefore, demonstrating calcifications can lead to errors in differential interpretation.

Some observers have relied on lobulations of a pancreatic mass and infiltration of the peripancreatic fat planes as indicators of malignancy.[8] However, these findings have also been observed in acute and chronic pancreatitis and are probably not specific.[10, 12, 14, 29, 31] The demonstration of retroperitoneal nodes or liver metastases with either modality certainly favors the diagnosis of a malignant process.

Finally, certain forms of chronic pancreatitis have been difficult to diagnose with either modality. On computed tomography, the gland may have a normal size and attenuation value. Similarly, the acoustical texture or size may appear normal on ultrasound. Atrophic forms of chronic pancreatitis may be similar to the normal fibrofatty infiltration that occurs with age on computed tomography. The increased echogenicity on ultrasound that accompanies these changes cannot always be distinguished from normal pancreas.

Conclusion

From this review of the initial experience with computed tomography and ultrasound, it is clear that both modalities have a major role to play in the noninvasive detection of pancreatic disease. Comparative studies with other noninvasive techniques have usually shown ultrasound or computed tomography to be more accurate.[1, 3, 34-36] However, neither computed tomography nor ultrasound has proved clearly superior to the other in all patients and in all pancreatic diseases. Limitations imposed by the types of energy utilized and existing instrumentation probably account for this finding. Fortunately, the strengths of one modality offset the weaknesses of the other such that one of the two techniques will be effective in most patients. Cost, risk and patient throughput considerations at the present time favor the use of ultrasound as the primary screening procedure. However, the final choice should be tailored to each patient.

In spite of the quantitation possible with computed tomography and the improved information content of contemporary ultrasonograms, the differential diagnosis of complex fluid abnormalities and solid masses is seldom possible. In some patients, the information provided by both modalities can lead to a more specific diagnosis.[23]

The therapeutic impact and effect on patient outcome resulting from the use of computed tomography and ultrasound is evolving. Clearly, the management of pseudocysts has been facilitated by both modalities.[25, 26] However, the earlier detection of pancreatic malignancy has not affected mortality figures.[37] On the other hand, the cost and morbidity associated with the diagnosis of pancreatic malignancies may be influenced by the use of computed tomography or ultrasound guided biopsies.[38-40]

Finally, it should be emphasized that some of the limitations presently observed with each modality are being eliminated by newer technology. Faster scanners capable of obtaining thinner sections, reconstruction in multiple planes, and newer contrast agents may improve the accuracy and differential diagnostic potential of computed tomography. Similarly, high-resolution real-time ultrasound systems and better quantitation of the data may improve the results with ultrasound. As technological advances are incorporated into each imaging system, additional re-evaluations will be necessary.

References

1. Haber K, Freimanis AK, Asher WM: Demonstration and dimensional analysis of the normal pancreas with gray scale echography. Am J Roentgenol 126:624–628, 1976.
2. Kreel L, Haertel M, Katz D: Computed tomography of the normal pancreas. J Computer Assisted Tomography 1:290–299, 1977.
3. Sample WF, Po JB, Gray RK, Cahill PJ: Gray scale ultrasonography: techniques in pancreatic scanning. Applied Radiology 4:63–67, 90–91, 1975.
4. Sample WF: Techniques for improved delineation of normal anatomy of the upper abdomen and high retroperitoneum with gray scale ultrasound. Radiology 124:197–202, 1977.
5. de Graaff CS, Taylor KJW, Simonds BD: Grey scale echography of the pancreas: re-evaluation of normal size. Radiology (In press).

6. Weill F, Schraub A, Eisenscher A, Bourgoin A: Ultrasonography of the normal pancreas. Radiology 123:417–423, 1977.
7. Moss AA, Kressel HY, Korobkin M, Goldberg HI, Rohlfing BM, Brasch RC: The effect of Gastrografin and Glucagon on CT scanning of the pancreas: a blind clinical trial. Radiology 126:711–714, 1978.
8. Kreel L: Computerized tomography of the pancreas. Computed Axial Tomography 1: 287–297, 1977.
9. Sample WF, Sarti DA: Computed body tomography and gray scale ultrasonography: anatomic correlations and pitfalls in the upper abdomen. Gastrointestinal Radiology (In press).
10. Sheedy PF, Stephens DH, Hattery RR, MacCarty RL: Computed tomography in the evaluation of patients with suspected carcinoma of the pancreas. Radiology 124:731–737, 1977.
11. Sheedy PF, Stephens DH, Hattery RR, MacCarty RL, Williamson B: Computed tomography in patients suspected of having carcinoma of the pancreas: recent experience. Presented at the 63rd Scientific Assembly of the Radiologic Society of North America, Chicago, IL, 1977.
12. Stanley RJ, Sagel SS, Levitt RG: Computed tomographic evaluation of the pancreas. Radiology 124:715–722, 1977.
13. Di Magno EP, Malagelada JR, Taylor WF, Go VLW: A prospective comparison of current diagnostic tests for pancreatic cancer. NEJM 297:737–742, 1977.
14. Ponette E, Pringot J, Baert AL, Marchal G, Dardenne AN, Coenen Y: Computerized tomography and ultrasonography in pancreatitis. Acta Gastro-Enterologica Belgica 39: 402–404, 1976.
15. Ferrucci JT, Wittenberg J, Black EB, Kirkpatrick RH, Schaffer D: CT findings in disorders of the pancreas. Exhibited at the 63rd Scientific Assembly of the Radiologic Society of North America, Chicago, IL, 1977.
16. Doust BD, Pearce JD: Gray scale ultrasonic properties of the normal and inflamed pancreas. Radiology 120:653–657, 1976.
17. Lawson TL: Sensitivity and specificity of pancreatic ultrasonography. Presented at the 63rd Scientific Assembly of the Radiologic Society of North America, Chicago, IL, 1977.
18. Leopold GR: Echographic study of the pancreas. JAMA 232:287–289, 1975.
19. Lutz H, Petzoldt R, Fuchs HF: Ultrasonic diagnosis of chronic pancreatitis. Acta Gastro-Enterologica Belgica 39:458–464, 1976.
20. Kazam E, Katz R, Herbstman C, Behan M: Computed tomography and ultrasonography of the pancreas: a comparative study. Presented at the 63rd Scientific Assembly of the Radiologic Society of North America, Chicago, IL, 1977.
21. Baker ML, Dalrymple GV: Biological effects of diagnostic ultrasound: a review. Radiology 126:479–483, 1978.
22. Fontana G, Bolondi L, Conti M, Plicchi G, Gullo L, Caletti GC, Labo G: An evaluation of echography in the diagnosis of pancreatic disease. Gut 17:228–234, 1976.
23. Carroll BA, Sample WF: Pancreatic Cystadenocarcinoma: CT body scan and grey scale ultrasound appearance. Am J Roentgenol (In press).
24. Kressel HY, Margulis AR, Godding GW, Filly RA, Moss AA, Korobkin M: CT scanning and ultrasound in the evaluation of pancreatic pseudocysts: a preliminary comparison. Radiology 126:153–157, 1978.
25. Leopold GR, Berk RN, Reinke RT: Echographic—radiological documentation of spontaneous rupture of a pancreatic pseudocyst into the duodenum. Radiology 102:699–700, 1972.
26. Sarti DA: Rapid development and spontaneous regression of pancreatic pseudocysts documented by ultrasound. Radiology 125:789–793, 1977.

27. Wolson AH, Walls WJ: Ultrasonic characteristics of cystadenoma of the pancreas. Radiology 119:203–205, 1976.
28. Fawcitt RA, Forbes WC, Isherwood I: Computed tomography in pancreatic disease. Br J Radiol 51:1–4, 1978.
29. Haaga JR, Alfidi RJ, Havrilla TR, Tubbs R, Gonzalez L, Meaney TF, Corsi MA: Definitive role of CT scanning of the pancreas. Radiology 124:723–730, 1977.
30. Levitt RG, Geisse GG, Sagel SS, Stanley RJ, Evens RG, Koehler RE, Jost RG: Complementary use of ultrasound and computed tomography in studies of the pancreas and kidney. Radiology 126:149–152, 1978.
31. Moss AA, Kressel HY: Computed tomography of the pancreas. Digestive Diseases 22: 1018–1027, 1977.
32. Gosink BB, Leopold GR: The dilated pancreatic duct: ultrasonic evaluation. Radiology 126:475–478, 1978.
33. Seidelmann FE, Cohen WN, Bryan PJ, Brown J: CT demonstration of the splenic vein–pancreatic relationship: the pseudo dilated pancreatic duct. Am J Roentgenol 129:17–21, 1977.
34. Barkin J, Vining D, Miale Jr, A, Gottlieb S, Redlhammer DE, Kalser MH: Computerized tomography, diagnostic ultrasound, and radionuclide scanning: comparison of efficacy in diagnosis of pancreatic carcinoma. JAMA 238:2040–2042, 1977.
35. Feinberg SB, Schreiber DR, Goodale R: Comparison of ultrasound pancreatic scanning and endoscopic retrograde cholangiopancreatograms: a retrospective study. J Clin Ultrasound 5:96–100, 1977.
36. Wood RAB, Moossa AR, Blackstone MO, Bowie J, Collins P, Lu CT: Comparative value of four methods of investigating the pancreas. Surgery 80:518–522, 1976.
37. McCormack LR, Seat SG, Strum WB: Pancreatic carcinoma: survival following detection by ultrasonic scanning. JAMA 238:240, 1977.
38. Haaga JR, Reich NE, Havrilla TR, Alfidi RJ, Meaney TF: CT guided biopsy. Cleveland Clinic Quarterly 44:1–7, 1977.
39. Hancke S, Holm HH, Koch F: Ultrasonically guided percutaneous fine needle biopsy of the pancreas. Surg Gynecol Obstet 140:361–364, 1975.
40. Smith EH, Bartrum RJ, Chang YC, D'Orsi CJ, Lokich J, Abbruzzese A, Dantono J: Percutaneous aspiration biopsy of the pancreas under ultrasonic guidance. NEJM 292: 825–828, 1975.

Anatomy and Pathology of the Biliary Tree as Demonstrated by Ultrasound

KENNETH J. W. TAYLOR
ARTHUR T. ROSENFIELD
CASPER S. DE GRAAFF

Since the commercial introduction of gray-scale machines in 1974, ultrasound has assumed an increasingly important role in the diagnosis of biliary tract disease. The initial 1974 report by Taylor and Carpenter[1] on ultrasonic visualization of dilated intrahepatic bile ducts in patients with surgical jaundice was supplemented by a report on the recognition of the common bile duct.[2, 3] These early observations have been confirmed by many others.[4-6] The clinical results of ultrasound in the differential diagnosis of jaundice are summarized below and the technique is now a well-recognized procedure wherever high quality ultrasound diagnostic facilities exist. However, despite the many criteria that have been described to aid recognition of the biliary tree, inexperienced ultrasonographers still report confusion between the dilated biliary tree and the dilated portal venous system. The anatomy of the normal and distended biliary tree is reviewed here. No single criterion provides reliable differentiation, but rather the combination of many characteristics that are seen on multiple tomographic sections. The technique for obtaining these sections is critical for their correct interpretation.

Scanning Techniques

The necessity for the development of compound scanning techniques as described by Donald et al in 1958,[7] was imposed by the limitations of the bistable equipment then available. Gray-scale equipment with amplification of nondirectional back-scattered echoes permits the use of simple linear and sector scans. The advantages of such simple scanning techniques over compounding were summarized by Taylor and Hill:[8]

1. The single registration of one reflector prevents degradation of resolution due to biological motion; compounding techniques lead to multiple registrations of the same reflector in many different positions during the respiratory and cardiac cycles.
2. In computing the distance of a reflector from the transducer based on the time of flight, assumptions must be made as to the velocity of sound in tissues. Different tissues have different sound velocities, which will lead to small inaccuracies in the geometrical placement of a reflector. This error will be compounded by multiple registrations in which the beam has passed through different tissues.
3. Accurate compounding depends upon absolute stability of the scanning arm, and some have therefore become unduly heavy to insure rigidity. Others show considerable degrees of slack, so that compounded scans will inevitably have severe degradation of resolution.
4. The resolution of ultrasound transducers is markedly better in the axial plane than in the lateral plane. Therefore, when single pass techniques are used, the axial resolution (about 1 mm) is retained. When scans are compounded, the poorer lateral resolution (3 – 10 mm) will occur in all planes.

Compound scanning techniques lead to degradation of resolution by biological motion as well as by other physical factors. Overwriting occuring due to compounding leads to the production of artifacts, destroys the shadowing behind gallstones, and makes reliable recognition of the dilated biliary tree impossible.

Scanning of the Biliary Tree

The patient is examined in a fasting state to obtain physiological dilatation of the gallbladder. The frequency used is 2.25 – 3.5 MHz in most adults, and 5 MHz in most children. The transducer is placed immediately below the xiphisternum, with the scanning arm arranged in the median plane. Using high gain, a slow paramedian scan is performed (Figure 1). Similar scans are made at least at every centimeter to the right and left of the midline. Oblique scans, with the scanning arm perpendicular to the costal margin, are particularly useful to display the cephalic portions of the portal vein (Figure 2). These scans are further supplemented by scans in the transverse plane. Again, simple scanning techniques are adequate. The scanning arm is arranged in the transverse plane, with the transducer placed immediately below the xiphisternum. During full inspiration, the transducer can be rotated from an acute angulation on one side to an acute position on the other side, producing a scan of about 160° (Figure 3). Multiple transverse sections can be taken at various distances below the xiphisternum, and when necessary the scanning arm can be angulated cephalically to visualize the liver substance underneath the hemidiaphragms. In a small number of patients, such subcostal scanning may be impossible, and intercostal scanning must be used. In such patients it

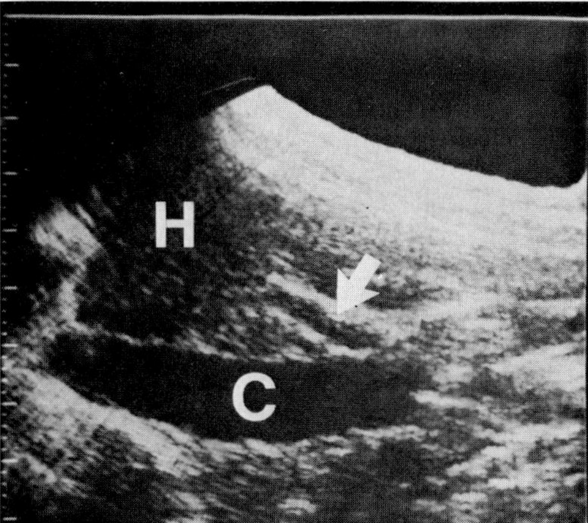

FIGURE 1. Parasagittal scan 2 cm to the right of the midline, showing the inferior vena cava (C), the lower portion of the portal vein (arrowed), and the liver (H).

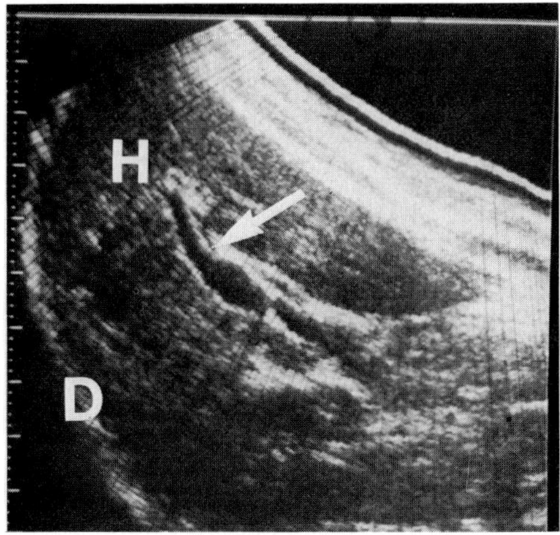

FIGURE 2. Oblique scan in a plane perpendicular to the right costal margin showing the cephalic portion of the portal vein (arrowed), the right lobe of the liver (H), and the right hemidiaphragm (D).

is advantageous to use a transducer with a 13 mm active face, placed in the intercostal spaces. Again, scans are performed in paramedial, oblique and transverse planes.

It must be stressed that the rigid scanning techniques described in many standard textbooks are to be deplored. If a patient is suspected of having gallstones, then multiple sections (between 50 and 100) must be taken in all planes through the gallbladder lumen in search of gallstones. The rigid observance of the 1 cm sections proposed in many textbooks may miss signifi-

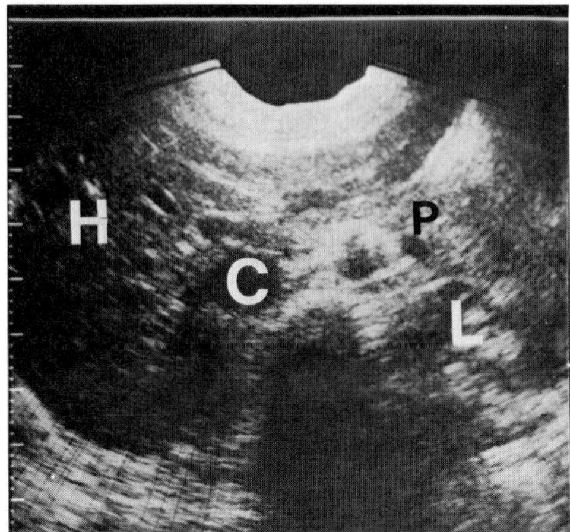

FIGURE 3. Transverse sector scan taken immediately below the xiphoid process. The right lobe of the liver (H) is seen. The inferior vena cava (C), the body and tail of the pancreas (P), and the left kidney (L) are also seen.

cant pathology. No protocol can substitute for properly trained technicians who are capable of interpreting the anatomy and pathology apparent on the scans and intelligently placing the next section based on that interpretation. Thus, if dilated ducts are seen, multiple sections are made to display the gallbladder, the entire biliary tree, the common bile duct, and the pancreas.

The Normal Biliary Tree

The Gallbladder

The gallbladder is well recognized in anatomy and pathology studies to be highly variable in its size, shape and anatomic location. Most commonly found in contact with the visceral surface of the right lobe of the liver, the gallbladder lies anterior to the right kidney (Figures 4a and b). However, the gallbladder may be on a mesentery or deeply embedded in the liver, and medial or more lateral locations are commonly seen. This type of anatomic variation imposes the need for flexibility during the examination. Since these patients are always examined fasting, the gallbladder lumen should be visualized. If it is not, either the patient has eaten, or the gallbladder is diseased and incapable of physiological distention, or there is congenital absence of the gallbladder. The incidence of congenital absence of the gallbladder is only 0.03 percent.[9] The most common cause of nonvisualization by ultrasound is disease which renders the walls incapable of physiologic distention. Of patients undergoing cholecystectomy, 12 percent have no lumen visible on ultrasound, but usually display high-level echoes and shadows in the region of the gallbladder fossa (Figure 5), suggesting a thickened gallbladder

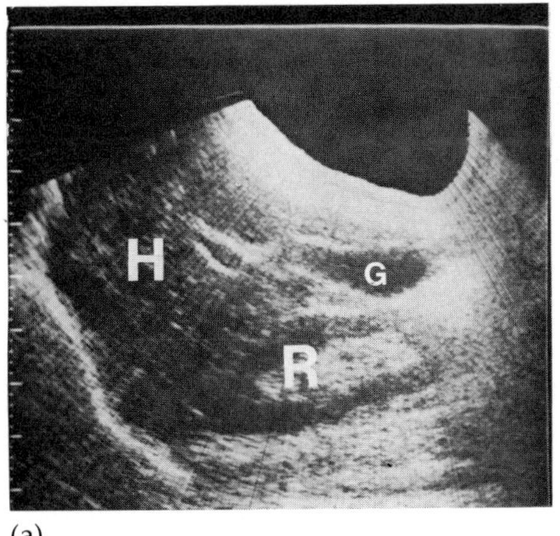

(a)

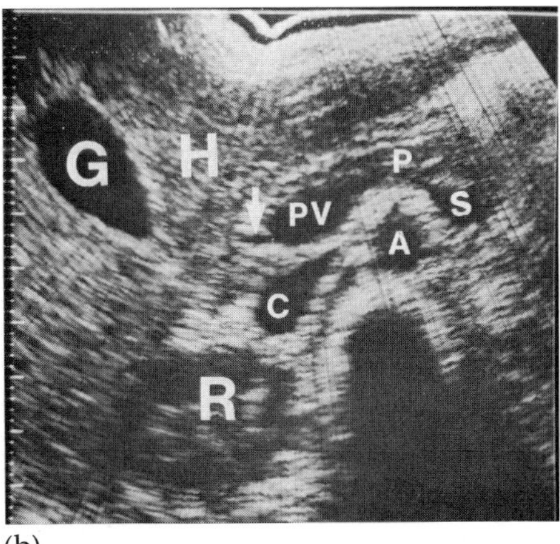

(b)

FIGURE 4. (a) Parasagittal scan through the right lobe of the liver (H) showing the gallbladder (G) lying anterior to the right kidney (R).

(b) Limited transverse scan through the right lobe of the liver (H). The lumen of the gallbladder (G), the right kidney (R), the inferior vena cava (C), the portal vein (PV), the splenic vein (S), the aorta (A), and the pancreas (P) are seen. The common bile duct (arrowed) is seen on the deep surface of the head of the pancreas.

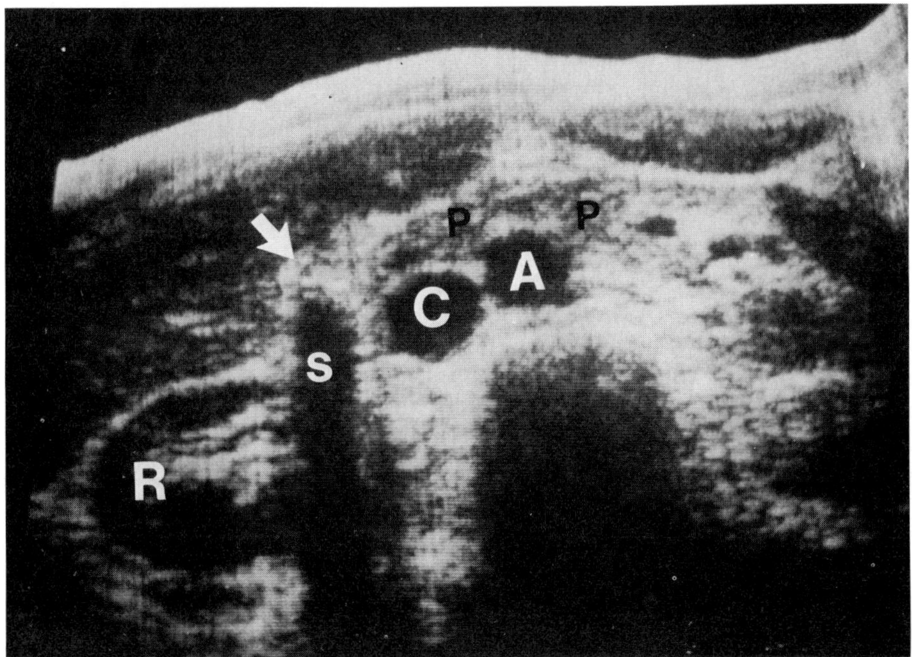

FIGURE 5. Transverse scan (compare with Figure 4b), showing the right kidney (R), inferior vena cava (C), aorta (A), and pancreas (P). Notice a highly-reflective mass (arrowed) with distal shadowing (S). These appearances are consistent with a small, contracted gallbladder full of gallstones.

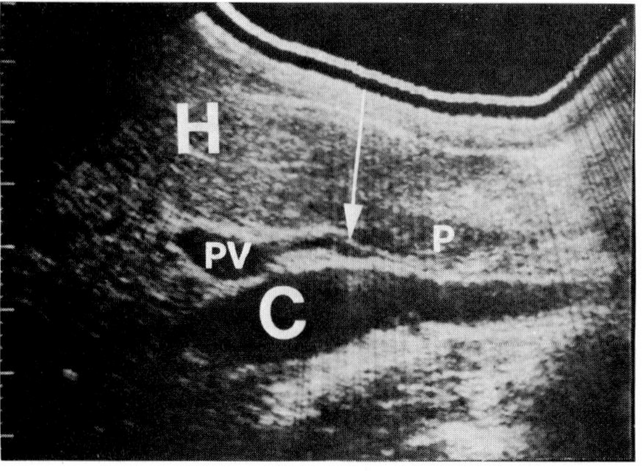

(a)

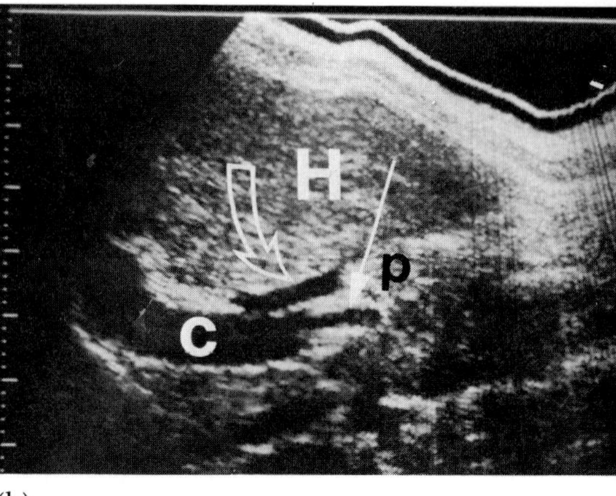

(b)

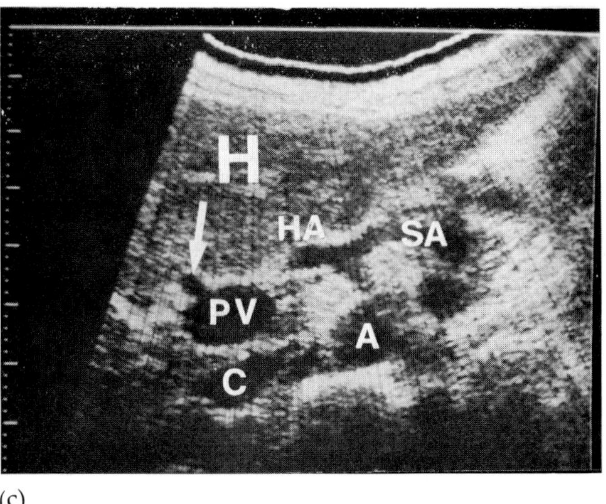

(c)

FIGURE 6. (a) Parasagittal ultrasonogram showing liver (H), inferior vena cava (C), the portal vein (PV), and the common bile duct (arrowed) passing deep to the head of the pancreas (P).

(b) Oblique longitudinal scan showing the liver (H), the inferior vena cava (C), the hepatic artery (open arrow), and the common bile duct (arrowed) passing deep to the head of the pancreas (p).

(c) High transverse scan showing inferior vena cava (C), the aorta (A), with the celiac trunk dividing into the hepatic artery (HA) and the splenic artery (SA). The portal vein (PV) is seen. A 4 mm tube (arrowed) immediately anterior to the portal vein is the common bile duct.

wall containing multiple gallstones.[10, 11] Thus, almost invariably, the nonvisualization of the gallbladder lumen on ultrasound examination indicates pathology.

The size of the gallbladder varies, both in the normal and abnormal organ. In our experience to date, no normal gallbladder has been found with a longitudinal axis exceeding 12 cm. However, many obstructed gallbladders are markedly smaller than this. The presence of a phrygian cap has been well documented by ultrasound.

The Biliary Canaliculi and Intrahepatic Bile Ducts

In the nondistended biliary tree the intrahepatic biliary canaliculi and ducts are seen but have a lumen of only about 1 mm on ultrasound examination (Figure 4b). There are two important sequelae of these observations made on many thousands of patients:

1. The normal biliary tree is essentially empty, with only a thin layer of bile separating the walls, and this fluid drains into the gallbladder or duodenum depending upon the activity of the sphincter of Oddi.
2. The presence of any dilatation of the intrahepatic biliary canaliculi, however minimal, must be regarded as pathological. Since the axial resolution of the ultrasound beam is 1 mm, any separation between the walls of the biliary tree exceeding 1 mm must be regarded as due to extrahepatic biliary obstruction. We have used this criterion for five years in thousands of patients referred with jaundice, and have had no false positive interpretations.

The Common Bile Duct

The normal common bile duct is seen on longitudinal section by taking multiple sections in the plane of the inferior vena cava. A very small tube, usually of approximately 4 mm diameter, is then seen passing deep to the head of the pancreas[12] (Figures 6a and b). Because of the angle between the interface and the ultrasound beam, the demarcation between the portal vein and the common bile duct is not usually displayed. On transverse scans (Figures 4b and 6c) the common bile duct is seen lying anterior to the portal vein on high sections and deep to the head of the pancreas on lower sections. Following cholecystectomy, the common bile duct is usually larger and appears to act as a temporary resevoir. Thus, in a post-cholecystectomy patient a dilated common bile duct is easily displayed (Figure 7), and is recognized as a tube running anterior to the portal vein and deep to the head of the pancreas.

Pathology of the Biliary Tree

The Gallbladder

The characteristic appearances of gallstones are described elsewhere in this issue (pp 128–132).

A suspected hydrops of the gallbladder is an important indication for ultrasound examination. Because of variations in the size and shape of the gallbladder, it is difficult to diagnose a hydrops on shape and size alone. How-

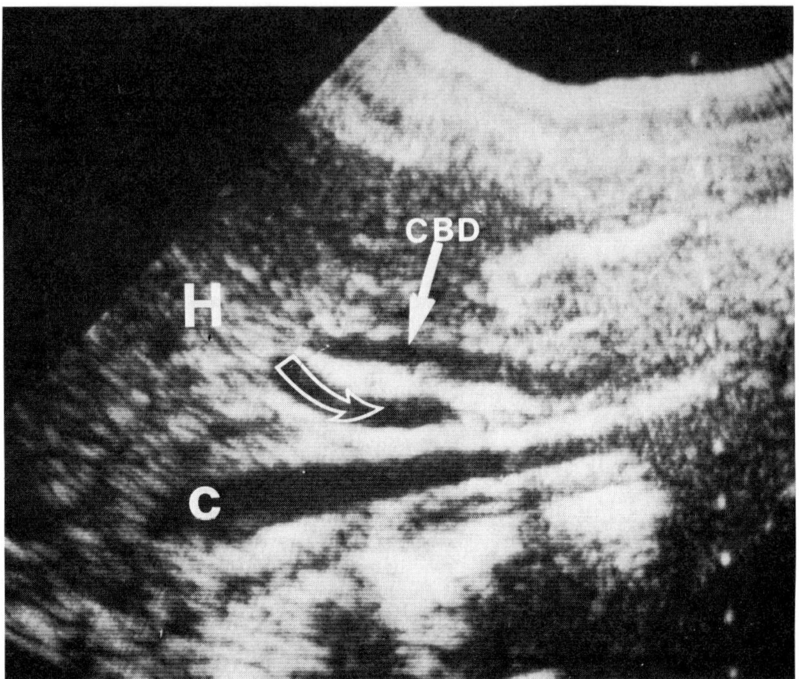

FIGURE 7. Parasagittal scan 2 cm to the right of the midline, showing the inferior vena cava (C) posterior to the liver (H). The portal vein (open arrow) and the distended common bile duct (CBD) are shown.

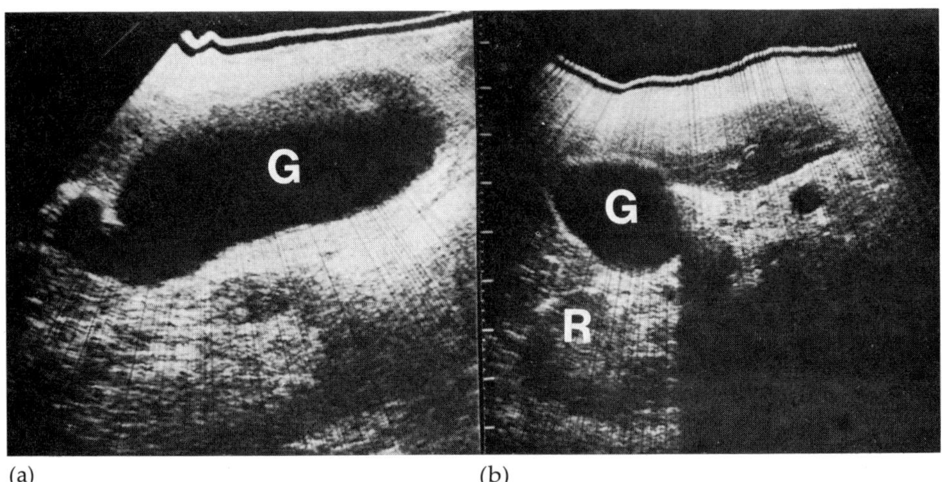

FIGURE 8. (a) Parasagittal ultrasonogram showing marked enlargement of the gallbladder lumen (G). The longitudinal axis measures 17 cm, which is far beyond the limits of normal.

(b) Transverse ultrasonogram showing hydrops of the gallbladder lumen (G). The right kidney (R) is seen posteriorly.

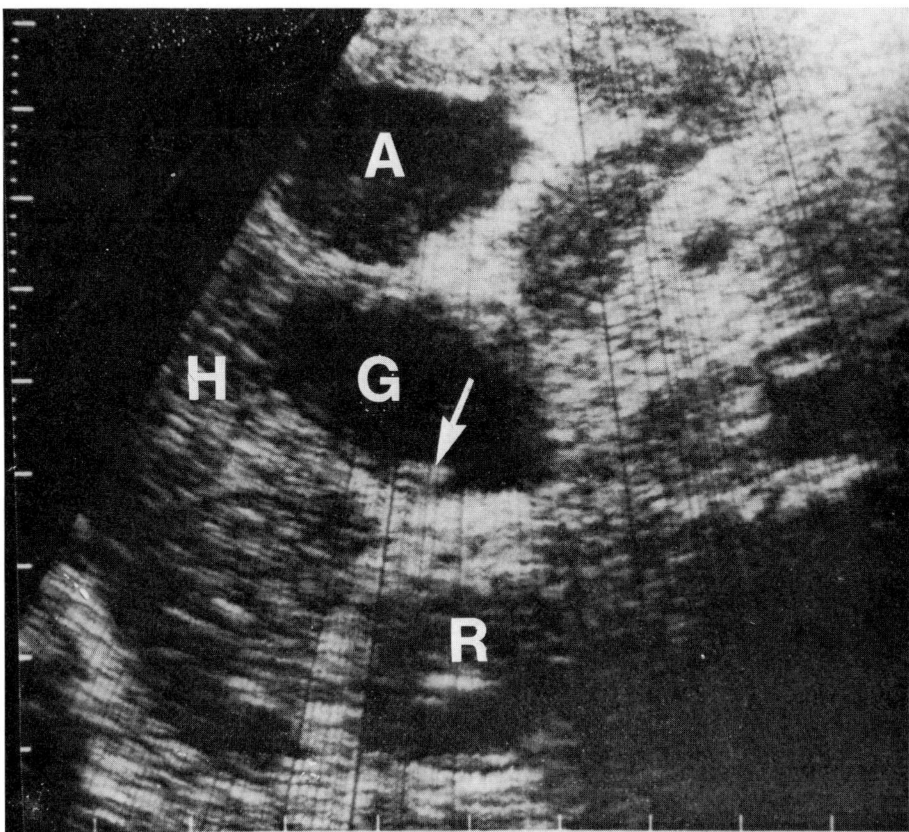

FIGURE 9. Transverse scan showing the lumen of the gallbladder (G). A gallstone within the lumen is arrowed. The right kidney (R) is seen posteriorly. The liver (H) is seen laterally. A further fluid-filled cavity (A) is seen anterior to the gallbladder, and this cavity contains some debris. These appearances are consistent with a pericholecystitic abscess secondary to perforation of the gallbladder.

ever, an obstructed gallbladder typically appears more spherical than one merely physiologically distended. When the longitudinal axis of the gallbladder exceeds 12 cm, physiological dilatation is unlikely. Figures 8a and 8b show marked dilatation of the gallbladder with the longitudinal axis of 17 cm which proved to be a hydrops. However, most hydropic gallbladders must be diagnosed by their failure to empty after a fatty meal or after cholecystokinin, or when the ultrasound examination is used in conjunction with clinical examination.

We have found little reliable correlation between thickening of the gallbladder wall and the condition at pathological follow-up. The wall appears thickened when ascites is present. This may be partly due to the signal processing, in that a large echo arising at a fluid—tissue interface and amplified

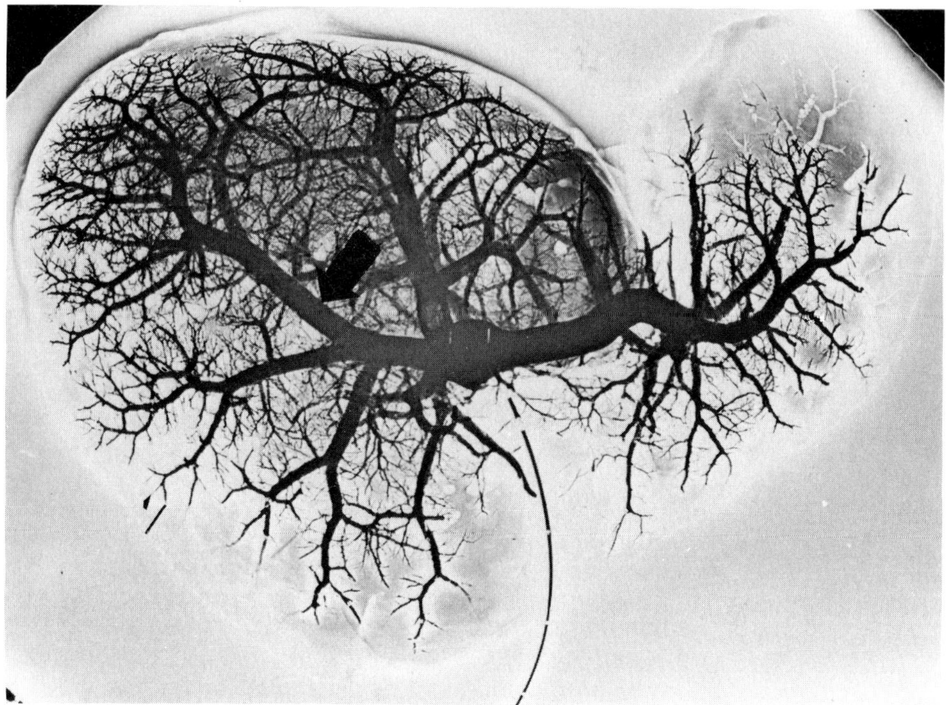

FIGURE 10. (a) Perfusion study of portal venous system. The right branch of the portal vein (arrowed) extends deeply into the right lobe of the liver, with minimal branching. Compare to Figure 11a. (Reprinted from *Ultrasound in Medicine*, ed. White DN, 4:125–134, 1978. With kind permission of Plenum Press.)

by passage through ascites in the presence of a normal time gain control (TGC) setting, results in very large echoes being modulated in size as well as brightness. Until signal processing is modified in all equipment to preclude such artifacts, we regard the thick-walled gallbladder as an unreliable sign of gallbladder pathology.

A pericholecystitic fluid collection can be an important finding of serious pathology. Figure 9 shows such a fluid collection lying within the liver substance, anterior to the gallbladder. The gallbladder contains a single stone and the appearances are consistent with an empyema of the gallbladder, with perforation and a surrounding abscess cavity.

The Dilated Biliary Tree in Comparison with the Portal Venous System

The diagnosis of a dilated biliary tree should not be made on the basis of a single tomogram. The condition is diagnosed by the appearances on multiple tomograms in both longitudinal and transverse planes, and by following the

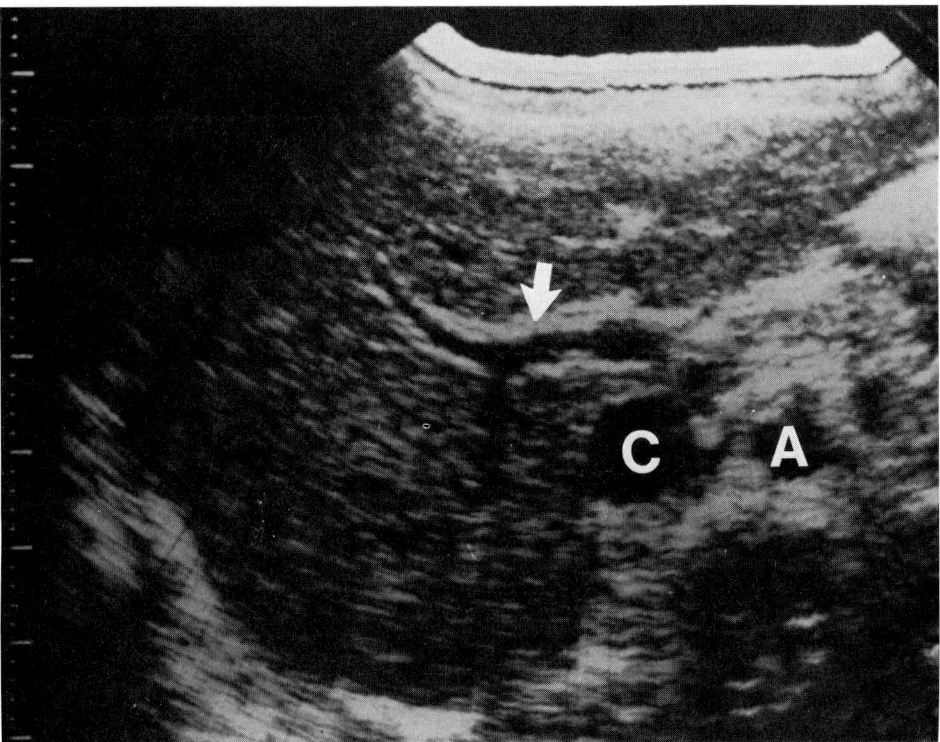

(b) Transverse scan through the liver, showing the right branch of the portal vein (arrowed) dividing distally into posterior and anterior branches. The inferior vena cava (C) and aorta (A) are seen posteriorly.

dilated vessels towards the porta hepatis into the portal vein or common bile duct. Certain characteristic appearances make possible reliable differentiation between venous distention and the dilated biliary tree. On transverse section, the right branch of the portal vein is seen as a vessel with highly reflective walls, which passes deeply into the right lobe of the liver before dividing into major anterior and posterior divisions (Figure 10a). This is in accord with the anatomy of the portal venous system as seen on injection studies (Figure 10b). The appearances of distal bifurcation of the portal venous system should be compared with those of the biliary tree, which are characterized by proximal bifurcation. Figure 11a shows an injection study of a post mortem liver. The biliary vessels are of similar caliber, with no significant decrease from proximal to distal, and there is proximal bifurcation of the major vessels. Thus, the transverse ultrasonogram (Figure 11b) shows the dilated biliary vessels spreading out like fingers from the region of the porta hepatis, in contrast to the portal venous system. As a result of this earlier and

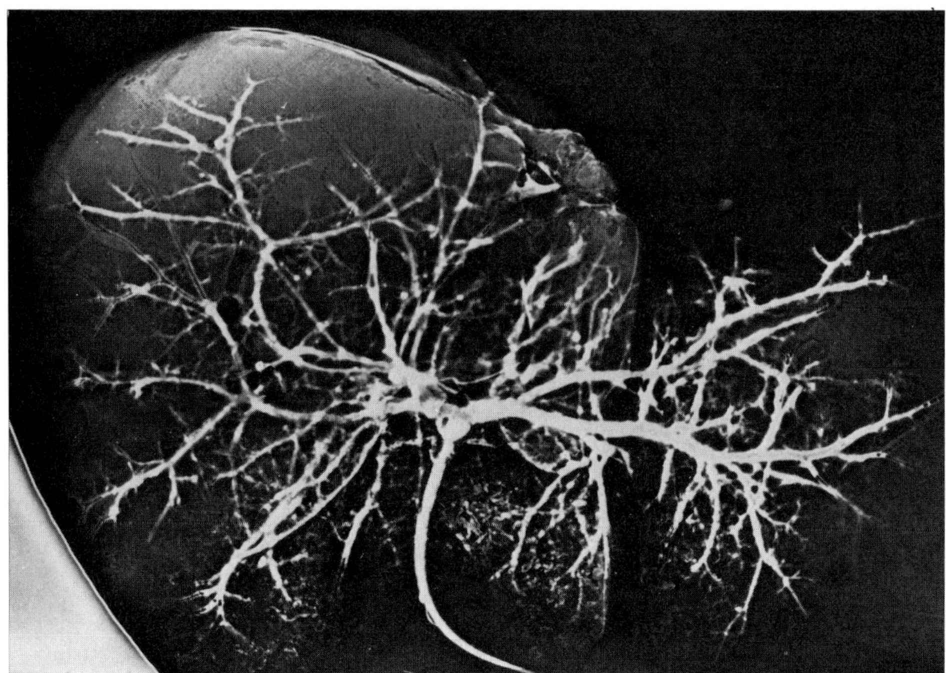

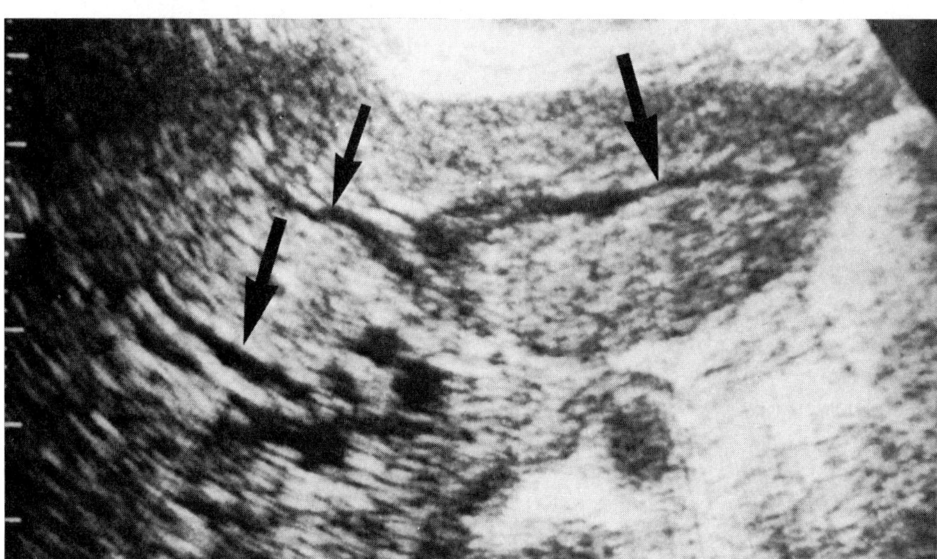

FIGURE 11. (a) Perfusion study of biliary tree, demonstrating early bifurcation of the biliary tree into multiple vessels of similar caliber. (Reprinted from *Ultrasound in Medicine*, ed. White DN, 4:125–134, 1978. With kind permission of Plenum Press.)

(b) Transverse scan of liver in extrahepatic biliary obstruction, showing multiple vessels (arrowed) of similar caliber extending out from the porta hepatis, due to proximal bifurcation of the biliary tree.

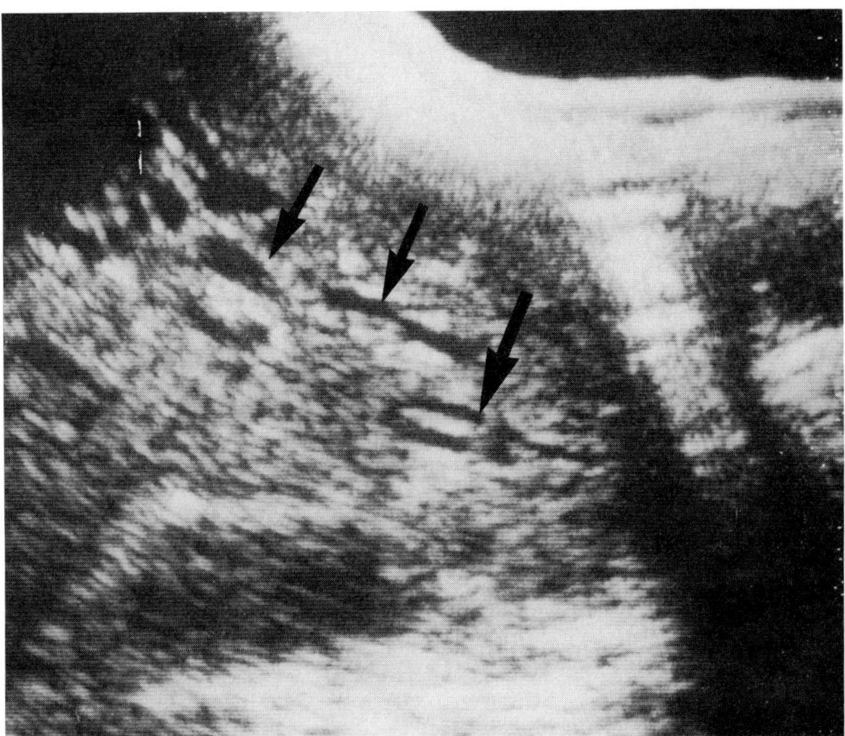

FIGURE 12. (a) Parasagittal ultrasonogram through the right lobe of the liver showing multiple dilated vessels (arrowed) which are approximately parallel to the skin surface. Note that only short segments of any one vessel are seen and these appearances are indicative of dilatation of the biliary canaliculi due to extrahepatic biliary obstruction. (Figure 12 continued over page)

more frequent bifurcation, multiple vessels are seen on any tomogram, whether in the transverse or longitudinal plane, and the typical appearances are as seen in Figure 12a. Multiple biliary vessels of similar caliber are seen parallel to the skin line or in a stellate configuration. Even in the most medial sections, multiple small but dilated biliary canaliculi are seen in extrahepatic obstruction (Figure 12b). Due to the extensive bifurcation of the biliary system only short segments of the biliary canaliculi are usually seen. When there is dilatation of the hepatic systemic venous system, much longer segments of the vessel are seen. Occasionally, stones are seen within the bile canaliculi.

The presence of a dilated common bile duct or dilatation of the gallbladder aids in the differentiation of the dilated biliary tree from the portal venous system. Techniques currently being developed, using a pulse Doppler device, help to differentiate vascular from nonvascular structures. Loh et al[13] demonstrated the clinical value of Doppler in identifying dilated biliary vessels as nonvascular structures. This was confirmed at this institution recently.[14]

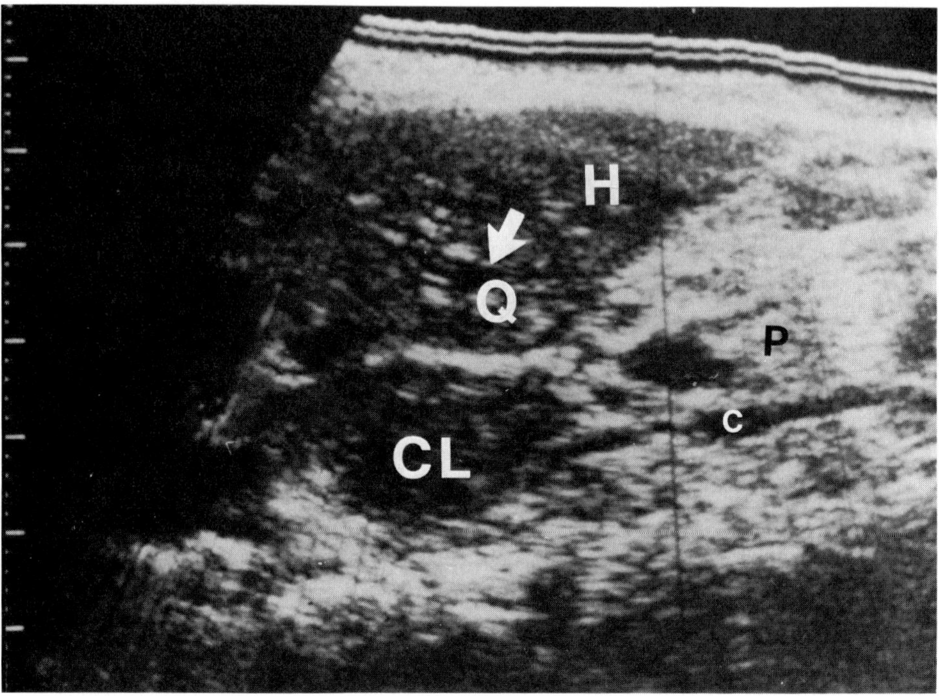

FIGURE 12 *continued.*

(b) Parasagittal scan 2 cm to the right of the midline. The inferior vena cava (C) is seen posterior to the pancreas (P), which is seen below the liver (H). The caudate lobe (CL) is seen posteriorly and the quadrate lobe (Q) anteriorly. Multiple small dilated channels are seen (arrowed). When air obscures the more lateral part of the liver, such near midline sections can almost always be obtained and suffice to make the diagnosis of extrahepatic biliary obstruction. These appearances are not mimicked by the venous system.

The Dilated Common Bile Duct

In a patient with a dilated intrahepatic biliary system every attempt should be made to visualize the common bile duct. Figure 13 shows the dilated duct lying anterior and almost parallel to the inferior vena cava, and the duct can be traced for 6 cm to an obstructing lesion in the region of the pancreas. Owing to intervening gas, the common bile duct can be seen in only 50 percent of patients with extrahepatic biliary obstruction.[4] Thus, although it is possible to predict an extrahepatic site of biliary obstruction, the precise anatomic site, in particular whether it is high or low obstruction, can be determined by ultrasound in only 50 percent of patients. Although common bile duct stones are frequently seen in distended common bile ducts, it should not be assumed that gallstones are the cause of the obstruction since they may occur in association with more sinister causes.

The manual scanning techniques described here, and currently required

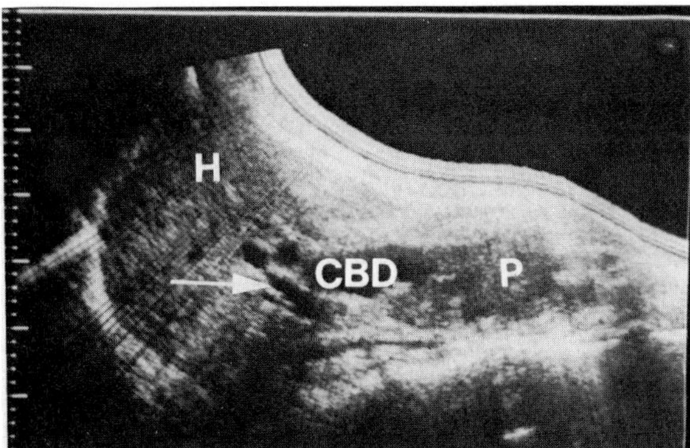

FIGURE 13. Parasagittal scan in the plane of the inferior vena cava. The portal vein is arrowed, and anteriorly the dilated common bile duct (CBD) can be seen running parallel to the inferior vena cava. A large pancreatic mass (P) is seen obstructing the distal end of the common bile duct. The liver is labelled H.

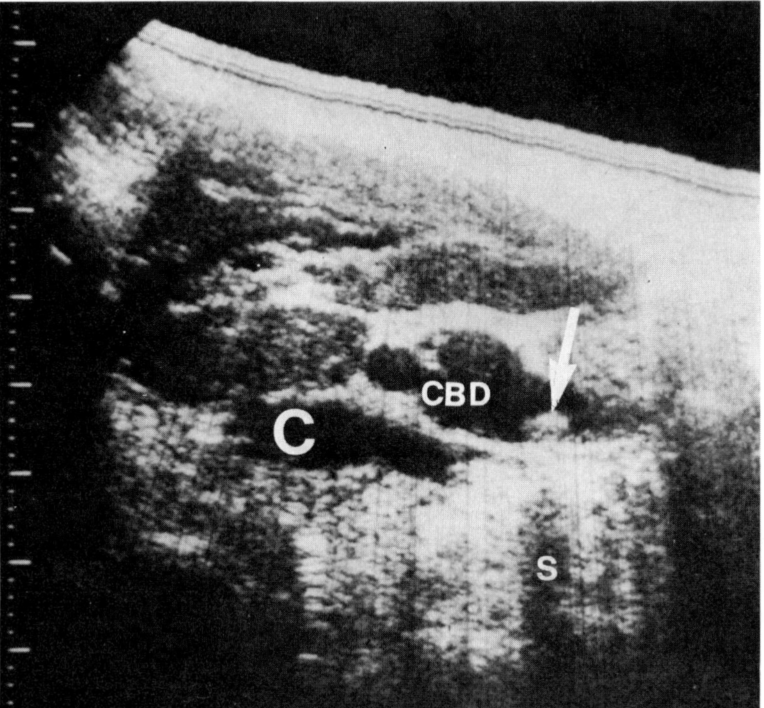

FIGURE 14. Parasagittal scan in the plane of the inferior vena cava (C). The common bile duct (CBD) is dilated and contains a definite stone (arrowed) which shadows distally. These appearances are diagnostic of a gallstone within the dilated bile duct. Despite these appearances, biliary obstruction was subclinical.

for high-quality gray-scale display, do not make ultrasound a suitable modality for reliably demonstrating common duct stones, for example after cholecystectomy. Ultrasound is a tomographic technique and small stones are easily missed. High resolution real-time systems may eventually be applied, but in our current experience, intravenous cholangiography is required to diagnose common duct stones accurately.

Acholuric Biliary Obstruction

The biliary tree may be dilated without clinical or biochemical evidence of jaundice. There are three conditions under which this phenomonon is seen in ultrasound scanning:

1. In patients with subclinical biliary obstruction, as in Figure 14. This patient had gross biliary dilatation, and multiple stones are seen within the biliary tree. She was not clinically jaundiced, nor was her serum bilirubin raised, presumably indicating only transient obstruction of the biliary tree associated with a ball-valve effect of the gallstones. More commonly this is seen in early carcinoma of the pancreas in which biliary tree dilatation is a response to subtotal biliary obstruction.
2. A dilated biliary tree may be seen unilaterally when there is obstruction to only one hepatic duct, as in Figure 15. This patient has dilatation of the biliary tree throughout the left lobe and there is evidence for a mass around the right branch of the portal vein. This highly reflective tumor suggests a sclerotic mass, such as a Klatskin tumor, obstructing the left hepatic duct. This was confirmed by skinny-needle biopsy which was ultrasonically directed.
3. After surgical relief of long-term obstruction to the biliary tree there may be persistent dilatation of the biliary tract. It is therefore important to elicit any previous history of extrahepatic biliary obstruction.

Clinical Results of the Diagnosis of Obstructive Jaundice and Observer Variability

Between 1973 and 1978 we followed up over 250 patients who presented with obstructive jaundice and had ultrasound examination. Using a dilated biliary tree as evidence of extrahepatic biliary obstruction, we observed dilatation in every patient with surgical jaundice, with one exception, and this was due to error in interpretation. False negatives do occur due to gallstones which produce transient dilatation of the biliary tree by a ball-valve effect. Thus, when the presence of dilated ducts was used to differentiate between intrahepatic and extrahepatic causes of biliary obstruction, an overall accuracy of 96.5 percent was achieved.[4] This accuracy depends upon observer experience.

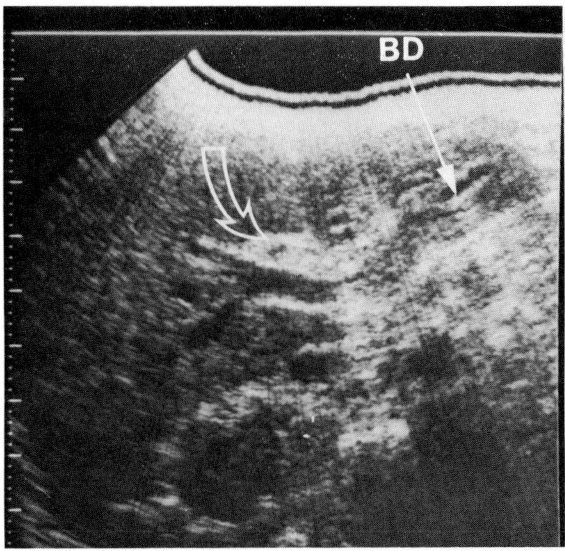

FIGURE 15. Transverse scan through the liver. Note that the left biliary tree is dilated (BD) whilst the biliary vessels throughout the right lobe of the liver are normal. There is a reflective mass around the walls of the portal vein (open arrow) which biopsy proved to be a cholangiocarcinoma obstructing the left hepatic duct. In view of the patent right hepatic duct, the patient was not jaundiced.

A group of physicians and one technician, of varied experience, read the ultrasound scans of 90 consecutive patients who had presented with jaundice. This reading was carried out blind and was repeated in two trials. The results, summarized in Table 1, showed the dependence on operator experience.[15] In particular they demonstrated the inadequacy of the one to three months which the average resident now spends in ultrasound training, and the greater inadequacy of the one-week courses which are the usual introduction to ultrasound for radiologists.

Conclusion

Gray-scale ultrasound techniques have opened up a wealth of anatomic and pathologic detail to the imaging specialist. In many patients suspected of having gallstones, ultrasound now represents the most accurate and the most rapid technique for diagnosis. Ultrasound is the most valuable technique in the immediate differential diagnosis of patients presenting with jaundice. For the vast majority of patients, it indicates whether they should proceed to early cholangiography and definitive surgery or, when the cause is intrahepatic, to biopsy or conservative treatment.

TABLE 1. Results of blind trials in diagnosis of obstructive jaundice.

Observer	Experience in Ultrasound	Trial 1 % Correct	Trial 2 % Correct
1. physician	>4 years	90	89
2. physician	<4 years	83	91
3. physician	2 years	83	89
4. technician	5 years	83	83
5. physician	5 months	75	83
6. physician	2 weeks	66	73

	Trial 1	Trial 2
False Positive Rate	7.95%	4.5%
False Negative Rate	6.8%	6.0%

We thank Plenum Press for permission to reprint Table 1, originally published in *Ultrasound in Medicine*, DN White, ed. 4:125–134, 1978.

References

1. Taylor KJW, Carpenter DA: Grey-scale ultrasonography in the investigation of obstructive jaundice (Letter to the Editor). Lancet, 2:586–587, 1974.
2. Taylor KJW, Carpenter DA, McCready VR: Ultrasound and scintigraphy in the differential diagnosis of obstructive jaundice. J Clin Ultrasound 2:105–116, 1974.
3. Goldberg BB: Ultrasonic cholangiography: Gray-scale B-scan evaluation of the common bile duct. Radiology 118:401–404, 1976.
4. Taylor KJW, Rosenfield AT: Grey-scale ultrasonography in the differential diagnosis of jaundice. Arch Surg 112:820–825, 1977.
5. Isikoff MB, Diaconis JN: Ultrasound: a new diagnostic approach to the jaundiced patient. J Am Med Assoc 238:221–223, 1977.
6. Neiman JL, Mintzer RA: Accuracy of biliary duct ultrasound: comparison with cholangiography. Am J Roentgenol 129:979–982, 1977.
7. Donald I, McVicar J, Brown TG: Investigation of abdominal masses by pulsed ultrasound. Lancet 1:1188–1194, 1958.
8. Taylor KJW, Hill CR: Scanning techniques in grey-scale ultrasonography. Br J Radiol 48: 918–920, 1975.
9. Monroe SE, Ragen FJ: Congenital absence of the gallbladder. CA Med 85:422–423, 1956.
10. Leopold G, Amberg J, Gosink BB, Mittelstaedt C: Gray-scale ultrasonic cholecystography: a comparison with conventional radiographic techniques. Radiol 121:445–448, 1976.
11. Crade M, Taylor KJW, Rosenfield AT, de Graaff CS, Minihan P: Surgical and pathological correlation of cholecystosonography (CCS) and cholecystography (OCG). Am J Roentgenol 131:227–230, 1978.
12. Sample WF: Techniques for improved delineation of normal anatomy of the upper abdomen and high retroperitoneum with gray-scale ultrasound. Radiol 124:197–202, 1977.
13. Loh CL, Atkinson P, Halliwell M: The differentiation of bile ducts and blood vessels using a pulse Doppler system. Ultrasound Med Biol (In press).

14. Taylor KJW, Atkinson P, de Graaff CS, Dembner AG, Rosenfield AT: Clinical evaluation of pulsed-Doppler device linked to grey-scale B-scan equipment, Radiology (In press).
15. Taylor KJW, Rosenfield AT, de Graaff CS, Simonds BD, Eckstein M, Moulton D, Wasson JFMcI: Factors affecting the recognition of the dilated biliary tree in the jaundiced patient. In Ultrasound in Medicine, ed. White DN; New York, Plenum Press, 4:125–134, 1978.

Comparison of Ultrasound and Oral Cholecystogram in the Diagnosis of Gallstones

MICHAEL CRADE

Gallbladder disease occurs frequently enough to justify the performance of over two million oral cholecystograms (OCG) annually.[1] Over 30 years of clinical use have made these images familiar, and the problems inherent in execution and interpretation are well recognized.

Gray-scale ultrasound is a new modality with images and techniques as yet unfamiliar to most physicians. Its tomographic nature mandates a precise knowledge of cross-sectional anatomy in transverse and longitudinal planes, and various oblique sections. Changes in anatomic relationships due to gravity and respiration must be understood. Versatile presentation is one of ultrasound's great advantages, but it also complicates orientation and interpretation.

Increasing evidence suggests that gray-scale ultrasound is the modality of choice for the accurate evaluation of many pathologic states. As a superficial fluid-filled sac, the gallbladder is perhaps an ideal organ for ultrasound evaluation. This paper details the current techniques and accuracy of ultrasound evaluation of the gallbladder, and compares it to the better known oral cholecystography.

Oral Cholecystogram

The oral cholecystogram has been one of the most trusted of radiologic procedures. Although it is said to be safe, accurate and relatively easy to perform, the various protocols proposed for film and pill taking probably reflect dissatisfaction more than scientific curiosity. Even the basic procedural routines remain controversial. Whether to give high or low fat diet,[2-4] exact scheduling of pill ingestion,[5] prior cleansing enema,[6] routine tomography,[7] first day vs second day examination,[8-11] "double dose" vs "single dose" are recurrent topics in the literature.

The accuracy of the OCG examination is reportedly high. In a study of 1207 patients, all with surgical confirmation, Baker and Hodgson found only 1.9 percent of their diagnoses to be in error.[12] Although others report similar impressive findings the true accuracy is difficult to evaluate[13, 14] because many problems cause poor absorption and the majority of patients with a poorly visualized gallbladder never come to surgery.[15]

For most patients with false normal OCG examinations, selective diet and serendipity will allow a life without biliary surgery or catastrophy. Others may progress to unfortunate complications. Caution in accepting the validity of a "normal study"[16] has been supported by numerous case reports.[17-20] White reported his series of 38 patients with "normal" OCGs but with recurrent symptoms. Thirty-four had gallstones at surgery, including 15 who suffered recurrent bouts of pancreatitis because of an inappropriate delay in therapy.[21] Some gastroenterologists have resorted to endoscopic bile drainage when the OCG is normal, yet their clinical suspicion of disease is high. Foss reported 70 such patients, surgically proving that 37 percent did indeed have significant gallbladder inflammation.[22]

Ultrasonic visualization of small, radiographically unsuspected, yet symptomatic stones has been reported.[23] In our series of 87 patients with both OCGs and ultrasonic examinations prior to finding stones at surgery there were six false normal OCGs (6.8 percent), all with positive ultrasound examinations. The accuracy of the OCG was found to be less than previously reported (93.2 percent vs 98 percent) and the usefulness of ultrasound was demonstrated.

When considering the reported accuracy of oral cholecystography, the selection of patients must be recalled; its application is not universal. The patient with acute cholecystitis may not be able to endure a diagnostic delay of one or possibly two days. Patients with nausea and vomiting will not effectively absorb the contrast, making the examination less than ideal. Patients with liver disease, pancreatitis, peritonitis, the traumatized and postoperative patient, and the very young, are not candidates for OCG,[24] and drug sensitivity or pregnancy may preclude the examination in other symptomatic patients. In one series, 14 percent of all patients actually undergoing OCG examination seemed to have such problems,[15] yet when accuracy is tabulated, they are simply excluded. It can be argued that this falsely elevates the OCG's reputed high degree of accuracy.

The OCG is a highly accurate procedure when it can be performed, but patients with jaundice or abdominal symptoms often attributable to gallstones simply are not candidates for OCG. Of the 151 patients in our series undergoing cholecystectomy, only 95 had had an OCG examination. This emphasizes the limited application of the OCG for many clinical situations, but also reflects growing acceptance of an ultrasonic diagnosis without radiographic confirmation.

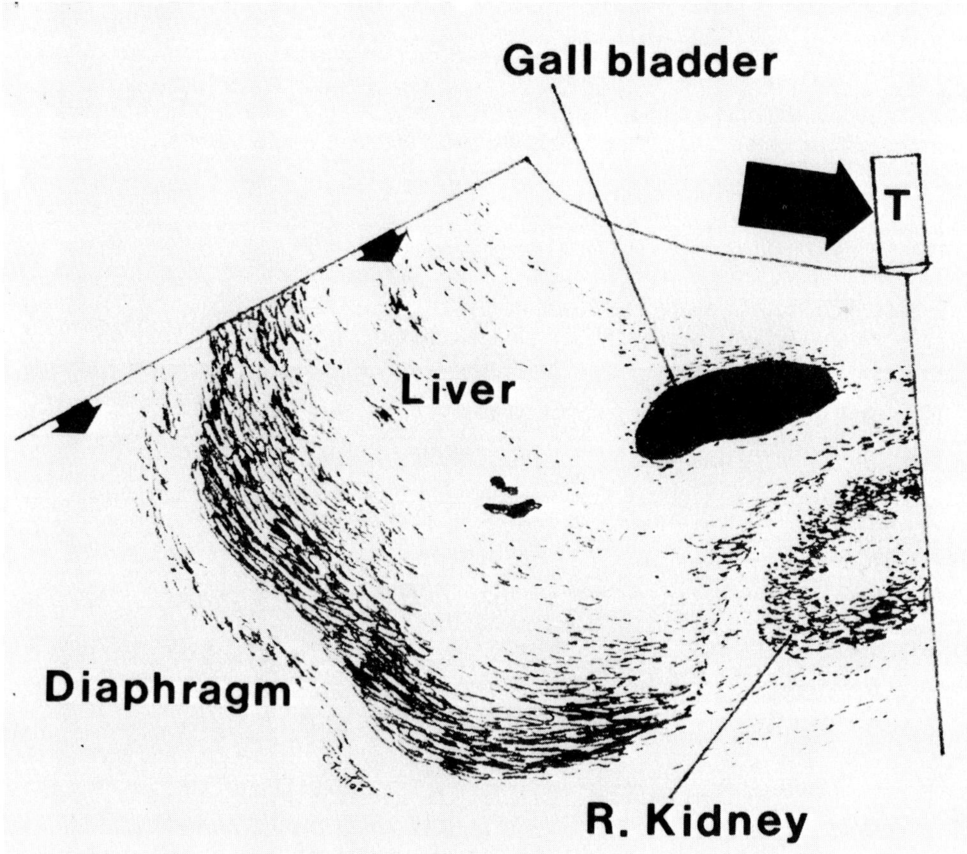

FIGURE 1. The gallbladder lumen embedded within the liver is best visualized by a single transducer (T) pass, using the overlying liver parenchyma as an acoustic window.

Ultrasound

As ultrasound technology improves, so too does its accuracy. Refinements in gray-scale instrumentation have clarified the bistable images so that abnormalities previously missed are now well defined.

Even with the newest units, however, improper setting, poor maintainance, shoddy technique, and careless documentation can totally erase all diagnostic advances. A high accuracy rate will be achieved by following this protocol:

1. Simple linear and sector scans of the area of interest should be used. Compounding may produce artifacts and obscure the distinguishing "shadow" of gallstones.
2. The overlying liver parenchyma should be used as an acoustic window as shown in Figure 1.

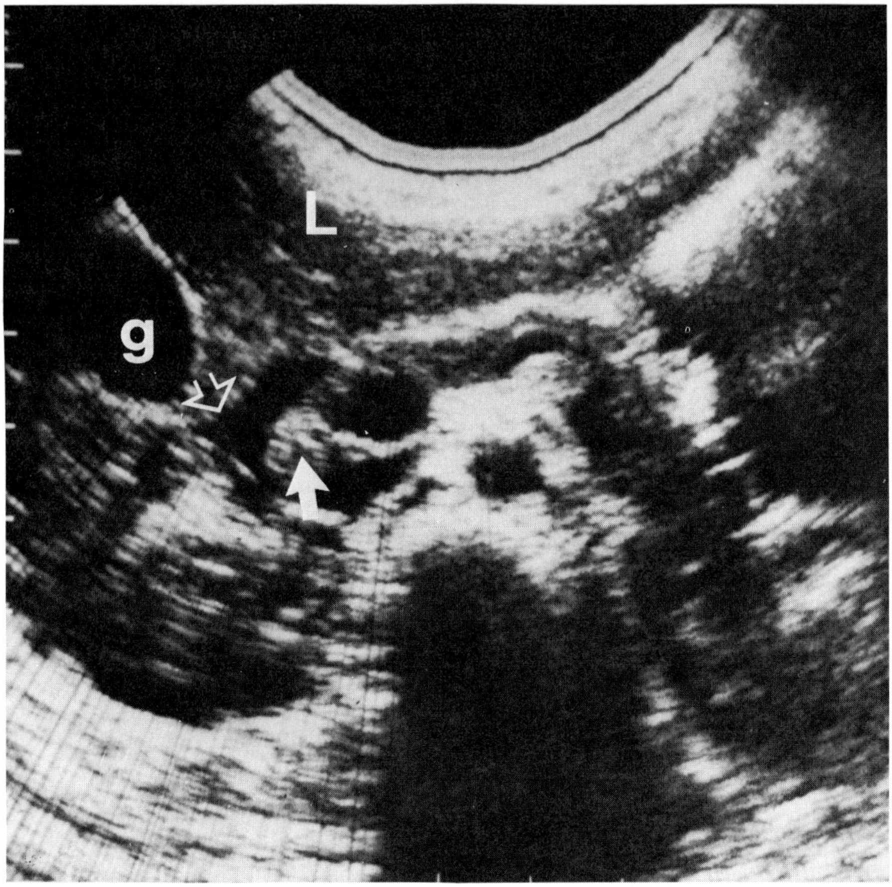

FIGURE 2. Transverse scan showing the normal gallbladder lumen (g) free of internal echoes, just lateral to the fluid-filled duodenum (open arrow) and the head of the pancreas (closed arrow). The liver parenchyma (L) is surrounding.

3. The gallbladder anatomy must be displayed in various planes and patient positions. Small stones in a large gallbladder may be difficult to find. Multiple tomographic sections are required to completely examine the gallbladder. The patient is scanned in the decubitus and erect positions: stones that collect together are more easily seen. The movement of intraluminal opacities should be documented.
4. The highest frequency that will penetrate the area of interest is used. In most adult patients a 3.5 MHz transducer, and possibly for the very thin or young patient a 5 MHz transducer, will provide the best images.
5. Patients are fasted for at least 6 hours prior to examination. The response of the normal gallbladder is to dilate; nonvisualization after fasting may indicate pathology. Most emergency patients have been on a self-imposed fast. If the lumen is not seen, the examination should be repeated during the next few hours of evaluation.

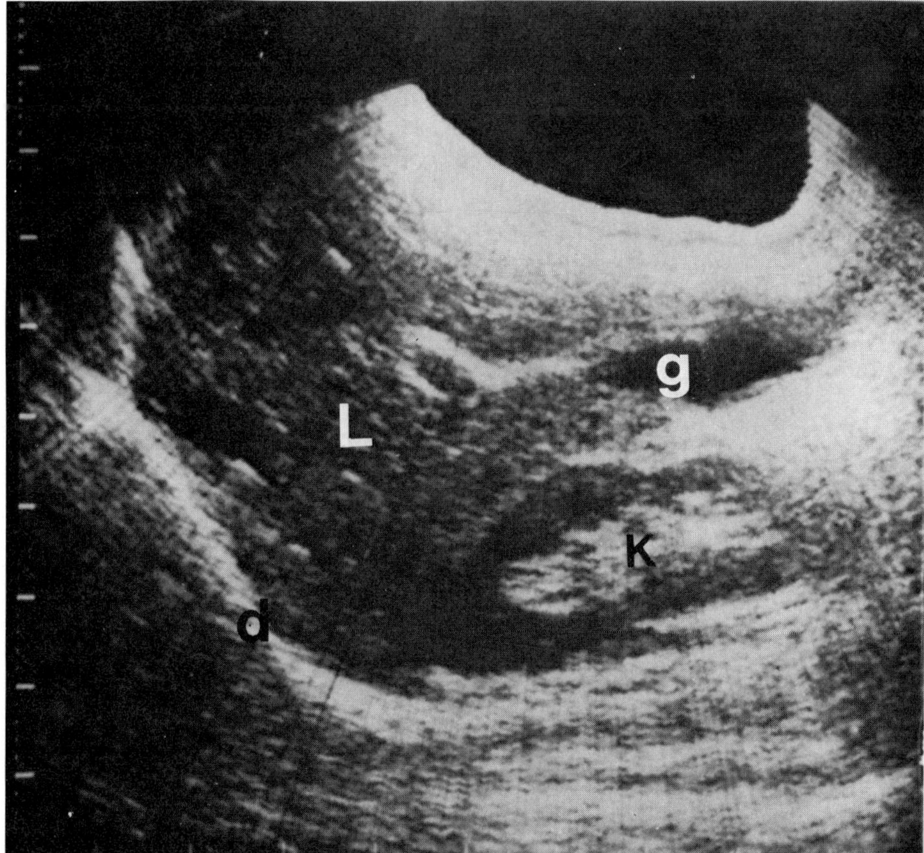

FIGURE 3. The echo-free lumen of the gallbladder (g) is seen just anterior to the kidney (K) in this normal longitudinal scan. Also demonstrated are diaphragm (d) and liver (L).

6. The abdomen should be physically examined. The radiologist should match visualized and palpated structures, correlating areas of tenderness with suspected scan abnormalities. Significant aspects of the symptoms and history should also be elicited.

By using such techniques, diagnostic accuracies of 91 percent[26] and 93 percent[27] have been reported.

The Normal Study

The normal gallbladder can be recognized easily as an oval, echo-free structure embedded in the medial and inferior aspects of the right lobe of the liver. In transverse section it lies just lateral to the duodenum (which may contain fluid, and at times displays shadowing due to mucus or food material), and lateral to the head of the pancreas (Figure 2). Typically it is seen anterior

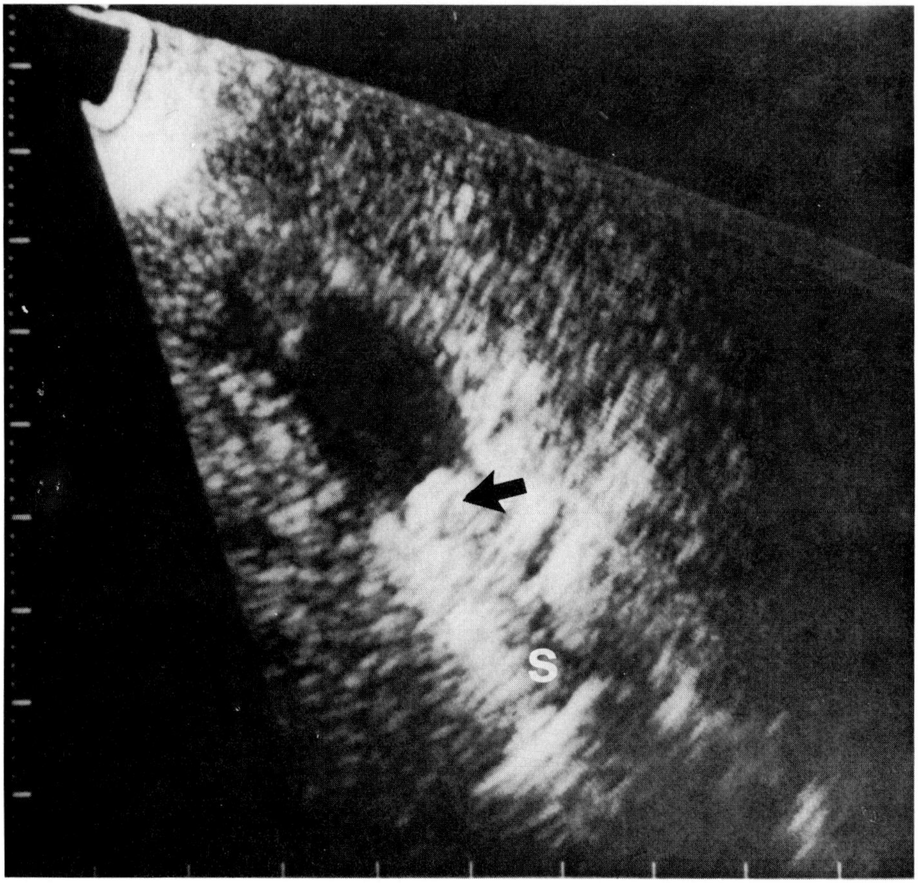

FIGURE 4. (a) Within the gallbladder is seen an opacity (arrowed) which shadows distally (S) and was subsequently shown to move with gravity. These findings satisfy Category I criteria and are virtually diagnostic of gallstones.

to the right kidney, and surrounded to some degree by liver parenchyma on longitudinal section (Figure 3).

The Abnormal Scan

After reviewing the hospital records of 151 consecutive patients who had had ultrasound prior to gallbladder surgery, three categories of scan abnormalities were established:

Category I: The presence of shadowing opacities which moved with gravity within a well defined gallbladder lumen (Figure 4a and b).

Category II: Ultrasonic nonvisualization of the gallbladder lumen, often with high-level echoes and shadowing in the area of the gallbladder fossa (Figure 5a and b).

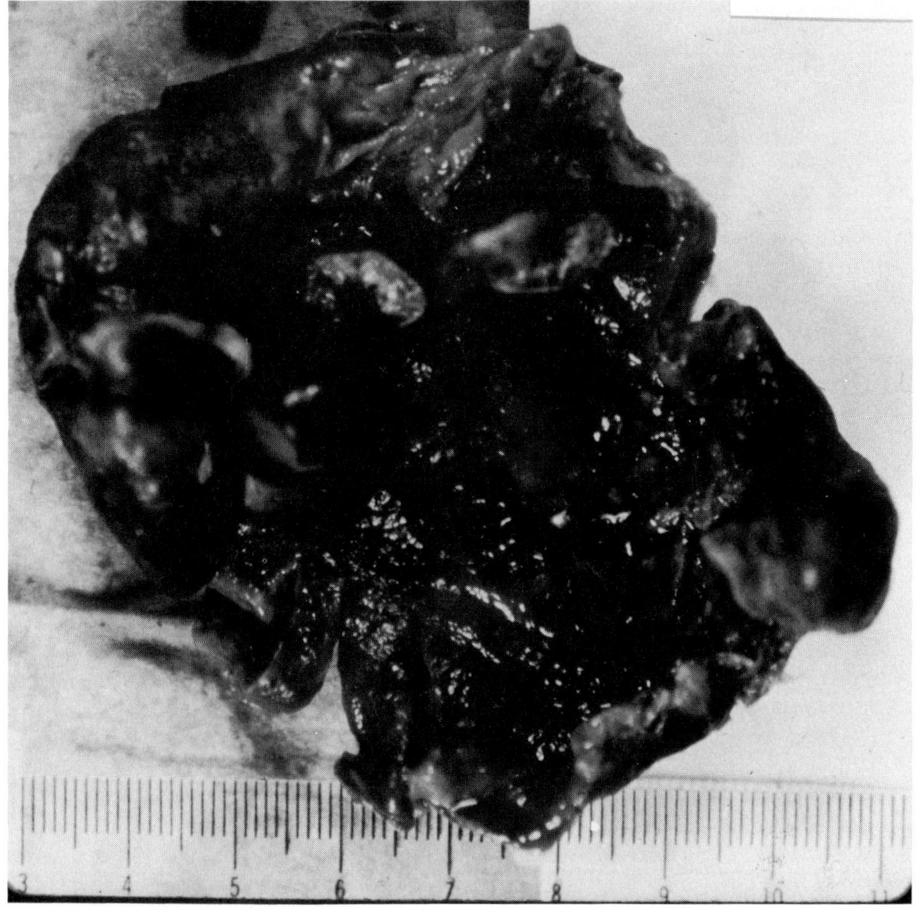

(b) Gallstones were subsequently found within an acutely inflamed gallbladder with a markedly thickened wall.

Category III: Non-shadowing opacities within the gallbladder lumen (Figure 6a and b).

Accuracy

Category I.

The classic appearance of gallstones, seen as intraluminal opacities which shadow distally and move with gravity, was found in 96 patients in our series. All 96 proved to have gallstones at surgery, giving an accuracy of 100 percent. One patient had an apparent intraluminal opacity that shadowed but did not move with gravity. Although at the time of the examination we felt this patient had gallstones, subsequent surgery found only a perforated

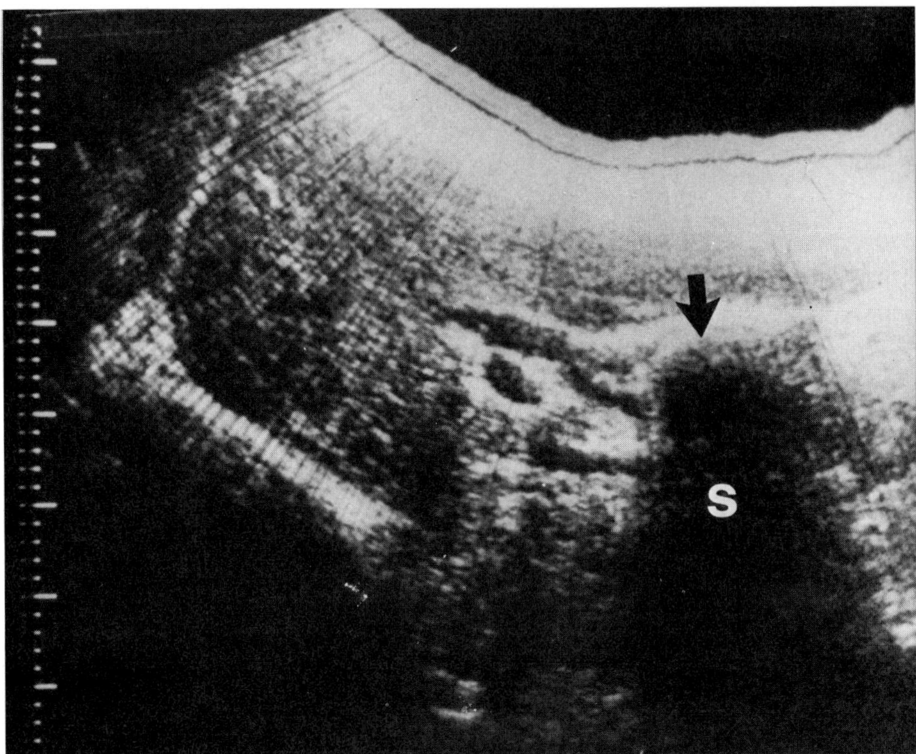

FIGURE 5. (a) High-level echoes (arrowed) with distal shadowing (S) are seen in the gallbladder fossa of a fasting patient. This longitudinal scan satisfies Category II requirements.

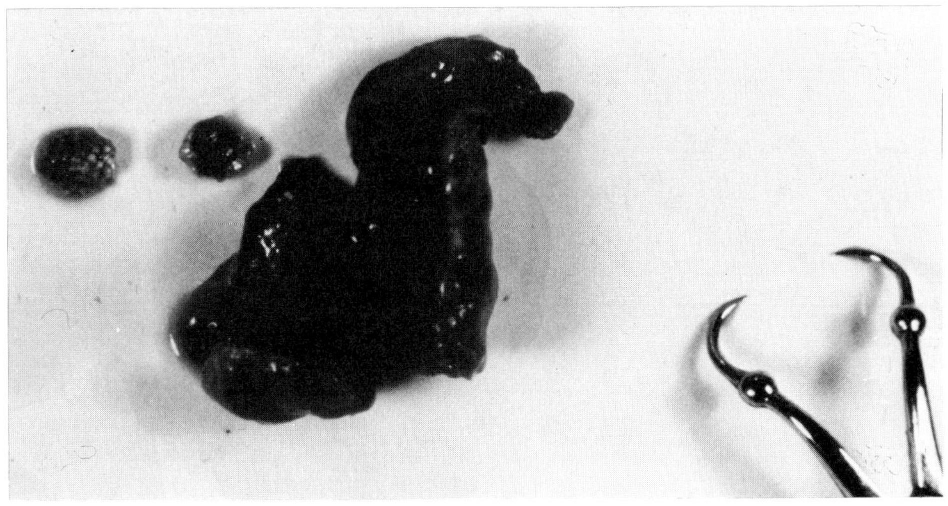

(b) A stone-containing gallbladder, shrunken by chronic inflammation was removed.

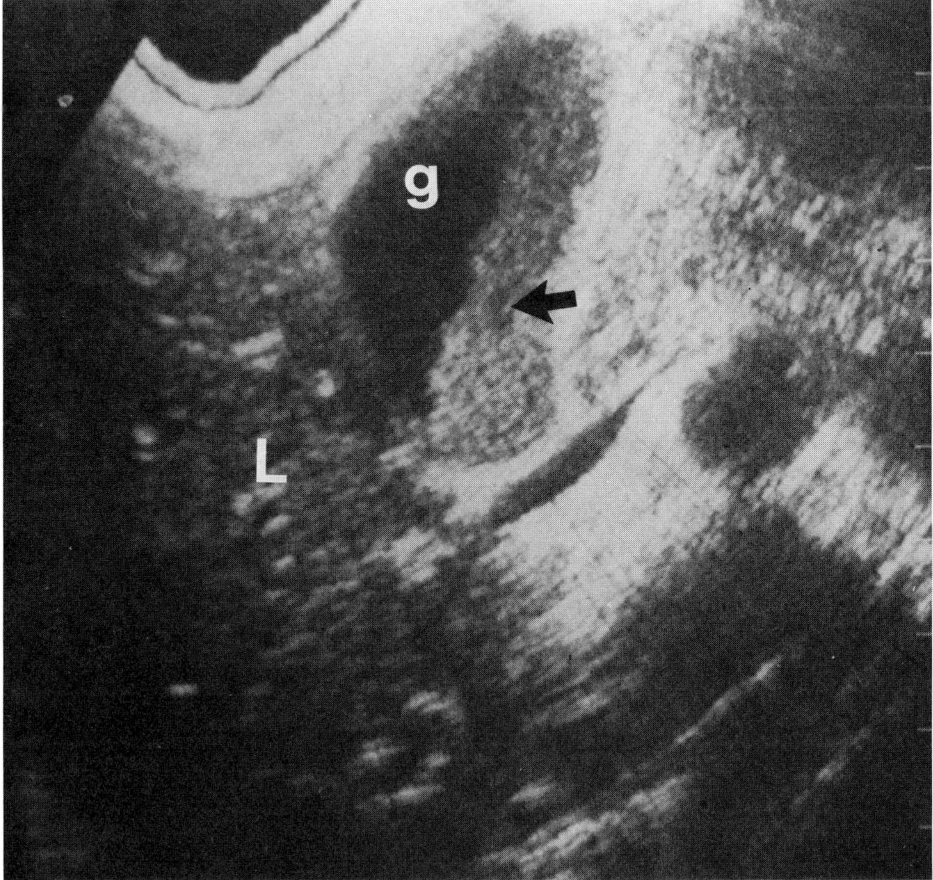

FIGURE 6. Category III criteria are demonstrated as multiple opacities (arrowed) which fail to shadow distally, within the gallbladder lumen (g). Liver is labelled (L).

duodenal ulcer, with inflammation and fibrosis surrounding the gallbladder fossa. Lacking documented opacity movement, this case does not fully meet Category I's criteria, and so is not included in our series. This experience illustrates that strict adherence to all criteria in each category is essential for reliable preoperative diagnosis. Of those patients with stones, the Category I pattern was seen in 70 percent.

Category II.

In 26 patients, there was no evidence of a gallbladder lumen, despite fasting and repeated examinations. High-level echoes with evidence of shadowing were sometimes seen within the gallbladder fossa. Twenty-five patients proved to have a shrunken, diseased gallbladder with gallstones. One patient (who also had the only normal OCG in this group) had no significant inflammation or gallstones at surgery. Because years of documented pain were relieved postoperatively, a tentative diagnosis of a dysergic gallbladder was suggested but a placebo effect may have occurred.

The overall accuracy of the ultrasound nonvisualized gallbladder was 96 percent (25 out of 26). This pattern occurred in 19 percent of those with proven stones. Careful scanning techniques are stressed, as similar opacities may occur from feces and air in the transverse colon, albeit in a different plane of section.

Category III.

A total of 18 patients had nonshadowing opacities within the gallbladder lumen. In each case, multiple scanning attempts, using varied transducer angles and machine outputs, failed to demonstrate distal shadowing. One patient who had had three normal OCGs was found at surgery to have a normal gallbladder, without inflammation or stones. The other 17 had significant inflammation. Eleven had stones, and six had acalculous cholecystitis, including one patient with a perforated gallbladder at the time of surgery. Of interest, two patients had quite large, single stones, measuring 4 cm × 2 cm and 3 cm × 2 cm. The reason for such nonshadowing is inexplicable at this time, although further study is underway.

The clinical significance of the Category III pattern is as yet unclear. Although only 61 percent of such patients proved to have gallstones, 94 percent had significant inflammation, thus justifying surgery. In one patient refusing surgery, serial scans disclosed a progression from normal to nonshadowing opacities (Category III), to a nonvisualized gallbladder (Category II). Almost certainly this patient had stones, and the phase of nonshadowing opacities represented an inflamed gallbladder on its way to stone formation. We therefore suggest that nonshadowing opacities, though not diagnostic of gallstones, may indicate an inflamed organ, possibly with lithogenic bile.

Other Signs of Abnormality

Others have reported an increased wall thickness as an ultrasonic clue to disease.[25] Although the thickened wall is pathologically a sign of chronic inflammation, no study has yet correlated specimens with ultrasound scans made prior to surgery. As of now, the "thickened wall" sign should not be relied upon alone for an abnormal diagnosis. Our series includes a case in which the wall was "thickened" on ultrasound, yet completely normal at pathology.

The gallbladder size is not as important as its shape. There is a great variation in size, some being large yet normal. When a round and tense appearance, not easily changed by transducer pressure is encountered, the possibility of hydrops of the gallbladder must be entertained.

Proven True/False Normals

Surgery confirmed the normal ultrasound for six patients in our study, including one pregnant 30 year-old thought to have cholecystitis, but proven to have had an intrahepatic abscess diagnosed by ultrasound (Figure 7). This

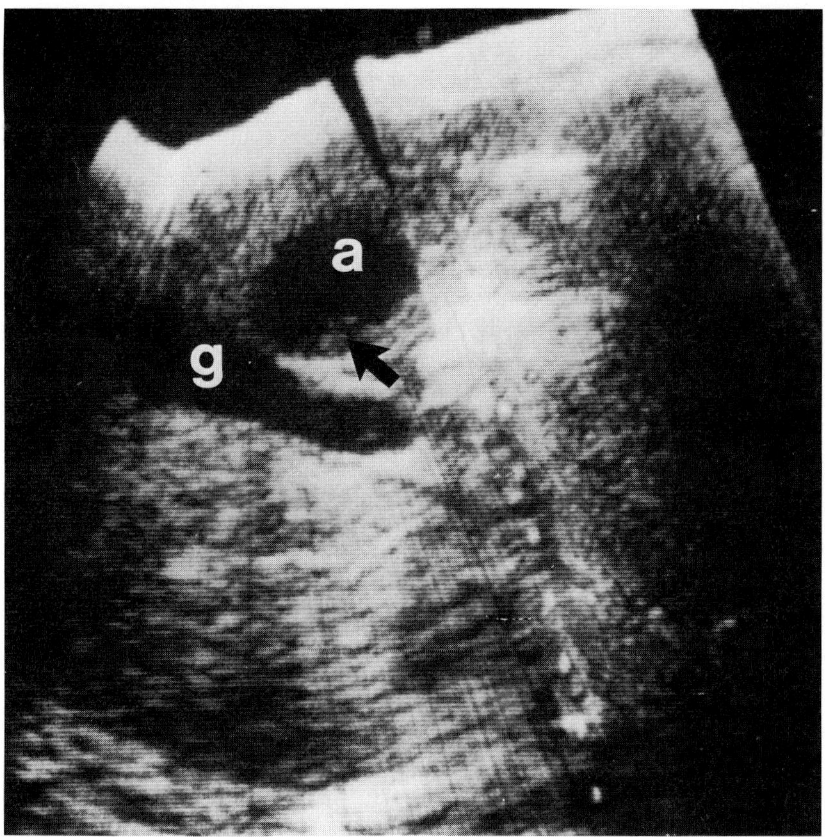

FIGURE 7. An abscess cavity (a) with settled debris (arrowed) is localized on this longitudinal scan. Adjacent to this cavity is the gallbladder (g) which was proven normal at surgery.

particular patient emphasizes the decided advantage of ultrasound in diagnosing clinically unsuspected disease, without the risks of radiation.

Five patients with normal scans proved to have gallstones at surgery. These errors were probably due to the tomographic technique, generating a false negative rate of 3 percent.

Discussion

It is difficult to overcome the inertia of already established routines. To do so there must be convincing advantages of accuracy as well as patient benefits. Ultrasound provides several such advantages:

1. Ultrasound can rapidly obtain a definitive diagnosis. Most examinations take no more than thirty minutes, unlike the one or two day OCG examination.

2. Ultrasound can benefit the emergency patient. The OCG can not.
3. Unsuspected disorders co-existing with gallbladder disease can be diagnosed by ultrasound. The OCG plays no diagnostic role in demonstrating a liver abscess or pancreatitis.
4. Patients are not refused ultrasonic evaluation because of problems of malabsorption, liver disease, peritonitis, etc. Such factors are all too important in selecting patients for OCG examination.
5. There are no drug or radiation hazards involved in ultrasound examination.

Although the OCG is currently the most widely used method for studying the gallbladder, it need not be used for all patients suspected of having cholecystitis. For those patients with ultrasound scans demonstrating shadowing opacities which move within the gallbladder lumen (Category I findings), the OCG need not be performed. The same is true for patients with high-level echoes in place of a physiologically dilated gallbladder after fasting (Category II). These scans account for over 88 percent of abnormal studies. Their high degree of accuracy (100 percent and 96 percent respectively), provides a very confident diagnosis of biliary tract disease.

When patients with Category III findings were brought to surgery, 94 percent proved to have significant cholecystitis, yet only 61 percent had stones. Because the number of such patients with only nonshadowing opacities within the gallbladder is small, we would continue to advise an OCG examination before surgical intervention.

We conclude, therefore, that ultrasound permits an accurate diagnosis of cholelithiasis and benefits especially those patients unsuited for OCG examination.

References

1. Burhenne HJ, Obata WG: The single visit oral cholecystography. New Engl J Med 292: 627, 1975.
2. Curl H: High fat diet preceding cholecystography: review of literature and experimental studies on filling normal gallbladder. J Am Med Assoc 119:607–610, 1942.
3. Mauthe H: The low fat meal in gallbladder examinations. Radiology 112:5–7, 1974.
4. Laufer I, Glendhile L: The value of the fatty meal in oral cholecystography. Radiology 114:525–527, 1975.
5. Koelher PR, Kyaw MM: Effect of fractionalized administration of Telepaque on gallbladder visualization. Radiology 108:517–519, 1973.
6. Shapiro JR, Stern W, Jacobson HG: Oral cholecystography: a review of techniques. Amer J Roentgenol 82:1003–1010, 1959.
7. Melnick GS, LoCurcio SB: The "nonvisualized" gallbladder: a tomographic re-evaluation. Radiology 108:513–515, 1973.
8. Berk R: The consecutive dose phenomenon in oral cholecystography. Amer J Roentgenol 110:230–234, 1970.

9. Mandelstam P: Cholecystography with iopanoic acid "reinforcement" before initial study. J Am Med Assoc 232:642, 1975.
10. Shopfner CE: Cholecystographic modification to improve initial study opacification (Letter to the Editor). J Am Med Assoc 234:479, 1975.
11. Wisoff CT: A comparative study of Telepaque dosage in cholecystography using single dose and double dose techniques. Virginia Med Month 87:88–90, 1960.
12. Baker HL, Hodgson JR: Oral cholecystography: an evaluation of its accuracy. Gastroenterology 34:1137–1145, 1958.
13. Beilin DS, Carlson GD: The clinical value of cholecystography by the oral method. Radiology 17:559–562, 1931.
14. Kerley P: The biliary tract. In Textbook of X-ray Diagnosis, eds. Shanks SC, Kerley P. Philadelphia, Sanders, 1958.
15. Mujahed A, Evans JA, Whalen JP: The non-opacified gallbladder on oral cholecystography. Radiology 112:1–3, 1974.
16. Farrar JR: Underdiagnosis of biliary tract disorders? Gastroenterology 51:1074–1075, 1966.
17. Kolodny M, Colker JL, Callahan EW, Baker WG Jr: Falsely negative cholecystography and cholangiography. Am J Dig Dis 13:669–673, 1968.
18. Case Records of Massachusetts General Hospital (Case #23, 1963): New Engl J Med 268: 731–735, 1963.
19. DeMuth WE Jr: Cholecystectomy following a normal cholecystogram. Am Surg 35:653, 1969.
20. Fiegenschuh WH, Loughry CW: The false normal oral cholecystogram. Surgery 81:239, 1977.
21. White T: Gallbladder stones with negative gallbladder X-rays. Am Surgeon 33:518–520, 1971.
22. Foss D, Laing R: Detection of gallbladder disease in patients with normal cholecystograms: results using a simplified biliary drainage technique. Dig Dis 22:685–689, 1977.
23. de Graaff CS, Dembner AG, Taylor KJW: Ultrasound and the false normal oral cholecystogram. Arch Surg 113:877–879, 1978.
24. Conquest HF, Spencer HS: Limitations of the oral cholecystogram. Virginia Med Month 92:527–535, 1965.
25. Leopold G, Amberg J, Gosink BB, Mittelstaedt C: Gray-scale ultrasonic cholecystography: a comparison with conventional radiographic techniques. Radiology 121: 445–448, 1976.
26. Bartrum R, Crow HC, Foote SR: Ultrasonic and radiographic cholecystography. New Engl J Med 296:538–541, 1977.

Percutaneous Aspiration and Biopsy Procedures under Ultrasound Visualization

HANS HENRIK HOLM
ORLA ALS
JENS GAMMELGAARD

Ultrasonically guided percutaneous puncture of organs and pathologic lesions was introduced in the early seventies. Using this technique it has proved possible to perform punctures for diagnostic and therapeutic purposes, especially in the abdomen.[1] The procedure is simple to perform, virtually without hazard, and causes very little discomfort to the patient.

This important new tool in the diagnostic armamentarium has numerous potential applications, and has already proved extremely useful. The method makes it possible to obtain material for cytologic, chemical, bacteriologic, histochemical and perhaps even immunologic studies from almost anywhere in the abdomen. Any organ or organ lesion that can be visualized on the ultrasound scan, can be subjected to puncture of fine needle aspiration biopsy. A widespread use of this technique can in many cases speed up the diagnostic evaluation of the patient, and short-circuit more expensive and less informative procedures. The general principles and indications described here are the ones used at the Herlev (previously Gentofte) Laboratory within the last few years.

Equipment and Methods

Puncture Guided by Manual Compound Scanning

A B-mode scanner equipped with a special puncture transducer is used. It is similar to the ordinary transducer except for a central canal in the axis of the

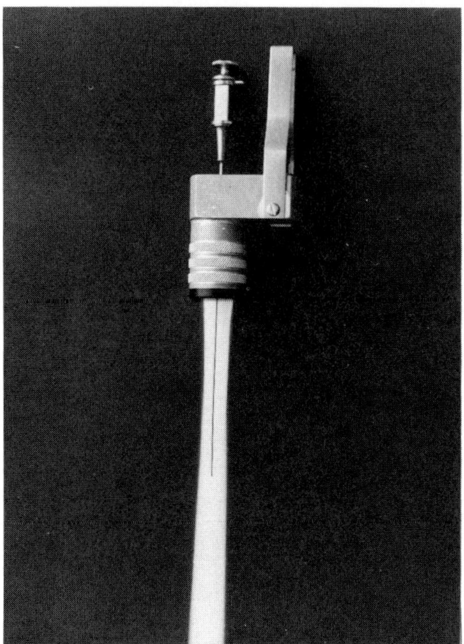

FIGURE 1. Aspiration needle in B-mode transducer. The puncture needle follows the sound beam emitted from the biopsy transducer.

transducer. A needle introduced through this canal will be guided in exactly the same direction as the sound beam emitted from the transducer (Figure 1). To allow sufficient room for needle manipulation the transducer is placed off-axis. The scanning arm system should be rigid, but light, without friction, and well-balanced in all positions. The canal in the puncture transducer should have a diameter (2.2 mm) sufficient for the passage of thick biopsy needles such as Menghini's or a Tru-Cut®. An adapter inserted in the central canal permits the use of needles with a smaller diameter.

Procedure

When a routine examination has disclosed the cystic or solid lesion to be punctured, the optimum plane and direction of puncture are selected and the site of the puncture is marked on the skin. The skin is then sterilized, local anesthetic is injected and sterile oil is applied. The puncture transducer, sterilized in a solution of Chlorhexidine, 5 percent for ten minutes, is mounted on the scanning arm and the area of interest is rescanned. The puncture transducer is placed at the site previously marked on the skin, and angulated until the beam visualized on the TV monitor by the electronic marker coincides with the desired needle pathway (Figure 2). The distance from the skin

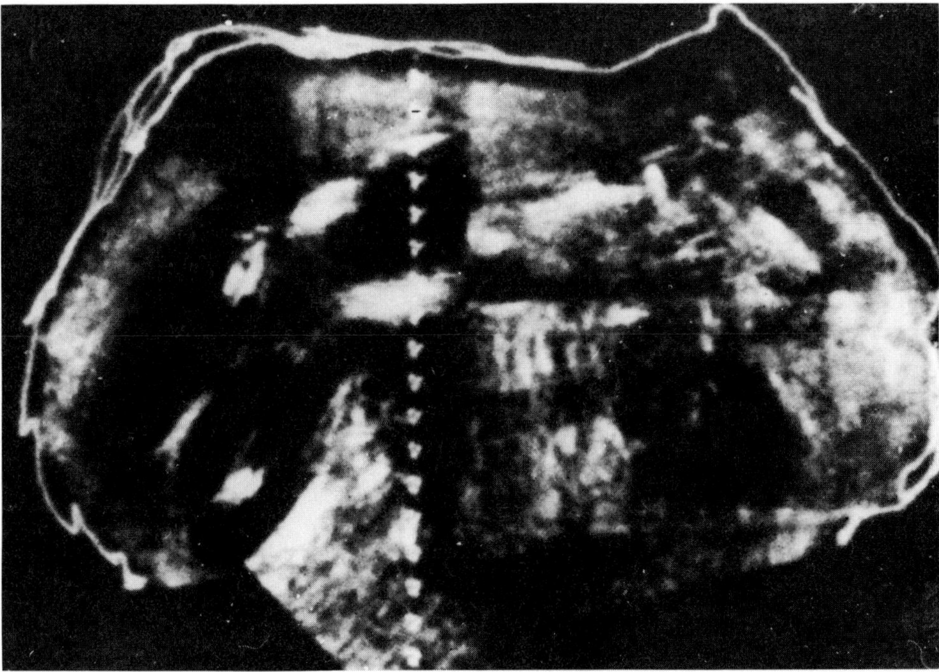

FIGURE 2. Transverse ultrasonogram showing tumor of the head of the pancreas. The desired needle pathway is marked at 1 cm intervals.

to the lesion is measured by the marker. This distance, plus the height of the puncture transducer, is marked on the needle with a set-screw to indicate the position of the needle-stop.

Puncture Guided by Dynamic (real-time) Scanning

A dynamic scanner is preferable when puncturing moving targets or performing amniocentesis and pericardiocentesis, because this type of scanner provides a live picture of the moving target. In many cases, especially when the lesion is cystic, the needle is visualized during its introduction (Figure 3). The canal for needle insertion has the same characteristics as described above and may be located centrally in the transducer array.

Procedure

The dynamic puncture transducer is moved over the area of interest until the optimal needle pathway as visualized on the image is seen to coincide with a perpendicular line on the monitor, corresponding to the direction of the puncture canal. An assistant may support the transducer in this position while the needle is introduced.

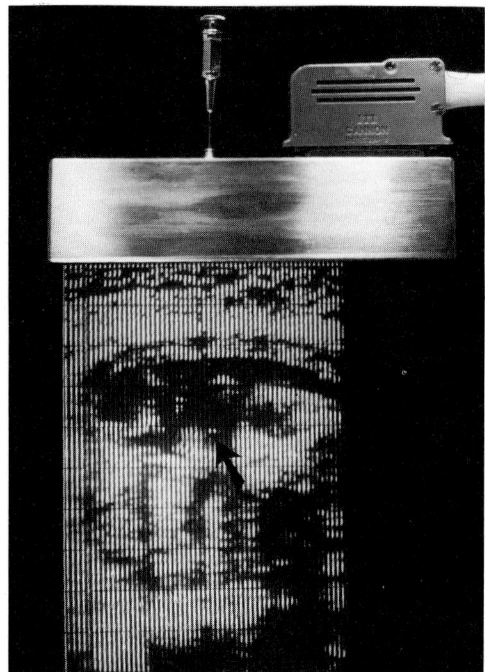

FIGURE 3. Linear array scan of gestation for aminocentesis. The echo from the needle tip is arrowed.

Needles used for Various Biopsy-Aspiration Procedures (Figure 4)

A. A thick needle (outer diameter 2.0 mm) like a Tru-Cut®, a Menghini or Iversen-Roholm, are advantageous in renal or liver biopsy, where a tissue core for histologic examination is desirable.
B. A 19-gauge needle (outer diameter 1.2 mm) is used for emptying fluid collections, and as an outer guide needle for the fine needle.
C. A 23-gauge needle (outer diameter 0.6 mm) is used for aspiration biopsy from suspected malignant solid lesions.

Several needle lengths are commercially available. The optimal length varies in each specific case, according to the location of the biopsy or puncture target.

Puncture of Cystic Lesions

Since the possibility of malignancy is very small and because emptying of the lesion is often desirable, a relatively large needle (1.2 mm) is used when puncturing fluid-filled lesions such as cysts, abscesses, hematomas and seromas. The needle is introduced to the predetermined depth and the fluid-filled lesion is emptied by aspiration with a sterile syringe (Figure 5).

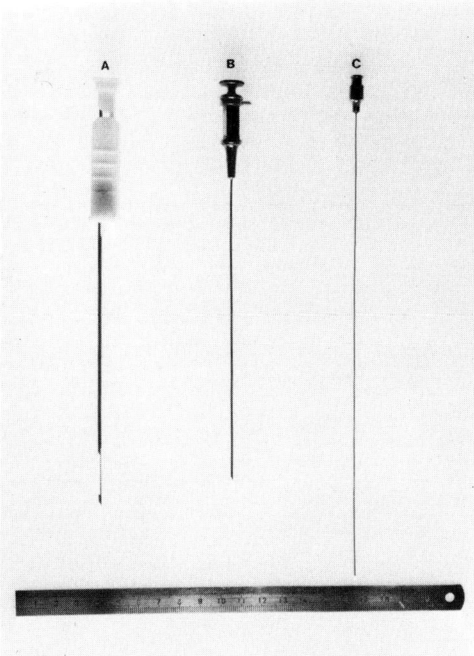

FIGURE 4. Different needles are used for different applications.
A. Biopsy needle (Tru-Cut®), outer diameter 2.0 mm.
B. Puncture needle, outer diameter 1.2 mm.
C. Aspiration biopsy needle, outer diameter 0.6 mm.

During puncture of echo-free lesions, it is often advantageous to watch the A-scope because:

1. The tip of the needle is visualized as a sharp echospike;
2. Possible respiratory movements of the lesion will be disclosed;
3. The collapse of the cyst wall is seen during aspiration.

The same information is readily obtained with a dynamic scanner, and it is a general trend at this laboratory that more punctures are performed with a dynamic multi-element puncture transducer.

The puncture technique described has been used in more than 1000 cases of renal cysts, pancreatic cysts, cystic liver lesions and various kinds of abdominal fluid collections such as abscesses and seromas. The main indications for puncturing cysts are to verify the diagnosis and to exclude the rare cases of malignancy. In the minority of cases the puncture proves to be therapeutic. For diagnostic purposes the fluid is sent for cytological examination and/or culture. However, its macroscopic appearance alone, such as blood, pus or clear yellow fluid, often gives sufficient information.

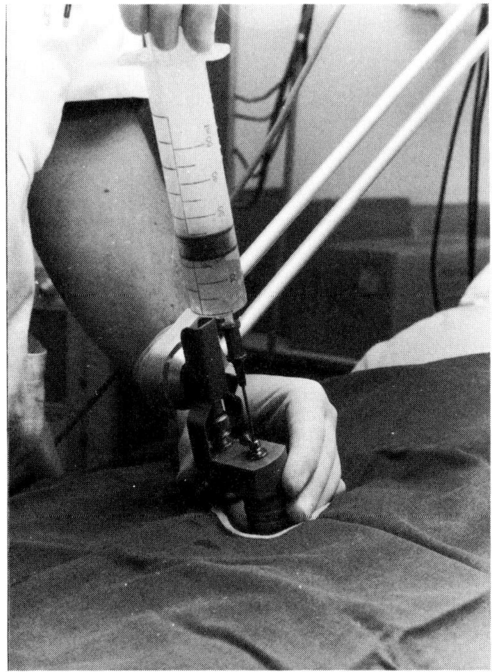

FIGURE 5. Puncture of cystic lesion. The fluid is aspirated directly into the syringe.

Ultrasonically Guided Nephrostomy

In patients with severely reduced renal function, both diagnosis and treatment may be a difficult clinical problem. Previously, emergency surgery was necessary if a postrenal obstruction was suspected and retrograde passage of a ureteral catheter was impossible. Under such circumstances an ultrasound examination is of great value, since the presence of a hydronephrosis can be diagnosed. When present, an ultrasonically guided nephrostomy using the Seldinger technique can be of considerable help.[2] A 14-gauge catheter with a curved tip introduced over a guide wire is used in most cases. The procedure has several advantages:

1. It is independent of renal function;
2. It relieves the hydronephrosis immediately in a most simple and atraumatic way;
3. Contrast injected through the catheter may lead to a radiographic identification of the site and nature of the obstruction.

Ultrasonically guided percutaneous nephrostomy using this technique has been attempted in 44 kidneys in the Herlev Laboratory. The etiology of the obstructive uropathies included ureteropelvic strictures and various cancers in the true pelvis. In 8 of the 44 kidneys the procedure was not successful because of the small size of the hydronephrosis, and in 6 cases the catheter slipped out unintentionally during the first 2 days. There were no complications.

Pregnancy

Amniocenteses in early pregnancy (i.e., 14–18 weeks) are performed to discover genetic abnormalities or to provoke abortion by injection of prostaglandin. When performed late in pregnancy, the lecithin/sphingomyelin ratio provides information concerning the maturity of the fetus. Before puncture, the fetus and placenta are outlined, minimizing the risk of complications. Guidance by real-time scanning is a great advantage because movements of the fetus can be detected.

Ultrasonically guided fetal injections of vitamin K have normalized the coagulation factors of the fetus prior to the birth in four cases where the mother had received anticoagulation therapy. Thus the severe risk of intracerebral hemorrhage is reduced.

Aspiration Biopsy of Solid Lesions

The scanning procedure is the same as described for cystic lesions. When a solid space-occupying lesion is disclosed there is always a high risk of malignancy. Thus, in the evaluation of solid abdominal masses such as focal liver lesions and pancreatic,[3] renal,[4] retroperitoneal or gynecological tumors, a fine needle aspiration biopsy technique is used, mainly to reduce or eliminate the risk of tumor-seeding.

An outer guide needle (1.2 mm diameter) introduced through the skin and immediate underlying tissue, should be used under these circumstances to ensure needle stability, to allow multiple passes of the fine needle and, finally, to avoid the spread of tumor cells.

The fine needle fitted to a 10 cc syringe attached to an aspiration handle, is introduced through the guide needle. When the tip of the fine needle is placed within the mass, the handle is retracted completely and the fine needle is moved back and forth in the tumor three or four times, continuously maintaining suction (Figure 6). When the aspiration is completed, it is important that the negative pressure in the system is equalized before the needle is withdrawn, to prevent contamination of cells from adjacent organs. After withdrawal, the syringe must be disconnected and filled with air, then reconnected and the material in the needle expelled onto glass slides. The fine needle aspiration may be repeated several times through the guide needle. The aspiration is made in various directions, from the center of the tumor and the periphery, to obtain representative material from all parts of the tumor.

During a fine needle aspiration it is often necessary to puncture through adjacent organs such as liver or parts of the gastrointestinal tract, and this can be done without any apparent harm. Prior to the liver and pancreatic punc-

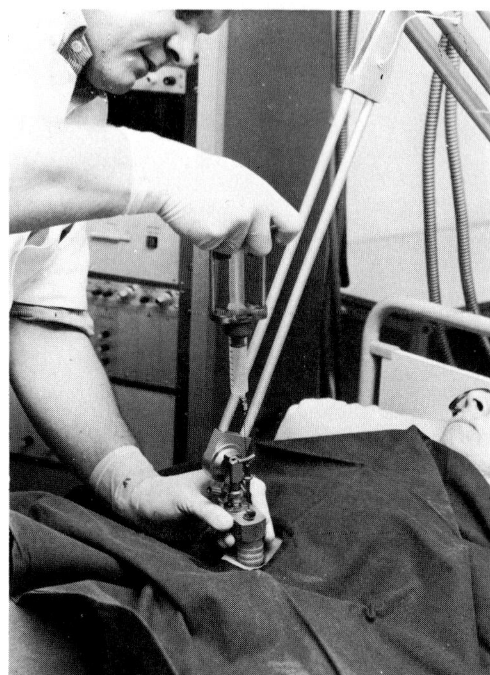

FIGURE 6. Aspiration biopsy of solid lesions. When the needle is inside the tumor, the aspiration handle is retracted completely. The outer guide needle allows multiple passages of the fine needle.

tures, a simple screening for clotting status is made, the patient having fasted. Franzen[5] has demonstrated that the vacuum obtainable with a 10 cc syringe is sufficient to obtain cell clusters in most cases.

Handling of the Aspirated Material

A single drop is expelled on each slide. The drop is spread over the slide with a single, gentle sweep in only one direction, using the edge of another slide. The specimen is thoroughly dried in the air, then fixed in methanol for 5 minutes before staining, for example by Giemsa technique.

Results

Pancreas

Ninety patients with suspected malignant lesions of the pancreas, later verified by surgery, autopsy or strong clinical evidence, were subjected to fine needle biopsy. Fifty-three proved to have carcinomas of the pancreas (Figure 7). When present the tumor cells were numerous and easily recognizable. In

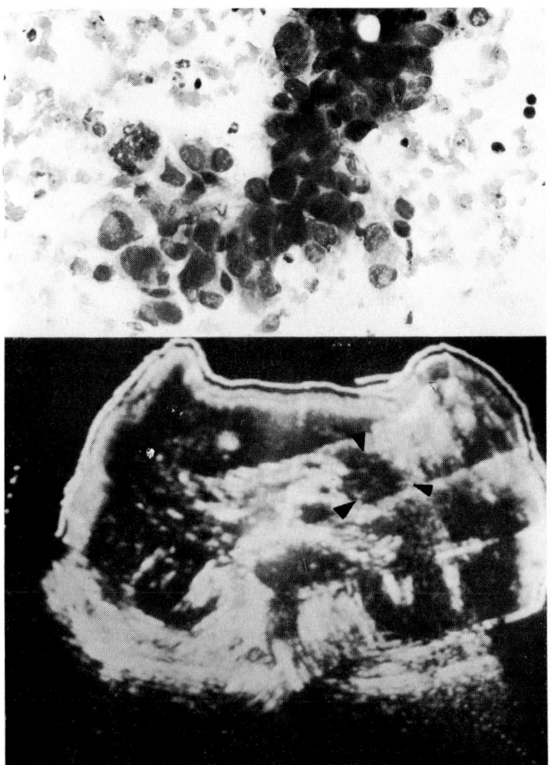

FIGURE 7. Solid tumor in the tail of the pancreas (arrowed). The cytologic specimen demonstrates malignant cells.

10 patients with pancreatic tumors, no malignant cells were aspirated despite an adequate aspirate. No malignant cells were aspirated in 35 out of 37 benign pancreatic lesions. In 2 cases the material was insufficient (Table 1). No false positive results occured, thus the pV_{pos} (predicted value of the positive) was 43/43 (100 percent). The pV_{neg} (predicted value of the negative) in this series was 35/45 (77.7 percent). A possible explanation for the pV_{neg} not being higher is that a carcinoma of the pancreas may be a small scirrhous tumor surrounded by relatively large amounts of inflammatory tissue from the aspirated area. This is in agreement with past experience which has found that the accuracy of surgical biopsy from a carcinoma of the pancreas does not exceed 85 percent.

The value of a precise diagnosis of a pancreatic lesion without surgery is obvious. With the technique described above, the early diagnosis of a carcinoma of the pancreas may be obtained in a patient with minimal symptoms. Furthermore, a laparotomy may be obviated when a malignant histology is obtained in a patient without jaundice, but with clinical or radiological evidence of inoperability.

TABLE 1. Pancreatic lesions—results of diagnosis by ultrasonically guided needle biopsy compared with final diagnosis.

			Cytologic Findings		
		Total	Malignant Cells	No Malignant Cells	Insufficient Material
Final Diagnosis	Malignant	53	43	10	0
	Benign	37	0	35	2
	Total	90	43	45	2

Kidneys

Fine needle biopsy was performed on 194 patients with suspected solid renal tumors. One hundred and forty-one proved to be carcinomas of the kidney, while 53 were benign lesions. The aspirated material revealed malignant cells in 119 of 141 patients (Figure 8). In 18 cases it did not, and in 4 cases the material was insufficient. No malignant cells were aspirated in 40 of the 53 benign kidney lesions, and in 6 cases the material was insufficient. There were 7 false positives (Table 2).

The pV_{pos} in these cases was 119/126 (94 percent). The pV_{neg} was only 40/58 (68.9 percent). The pV_{pos} is strained by 7 false positives. In 2 cases, surgery following the biopsy procedure revealed benign cysts and, in 3 cases, inflammatory processes. In the last 2 cases small adenomas were discovered in the renal parenchyma, and it is known that the cytologic material from an adenoma, and that from a highly differentiated carcinoma of the kidney are indistinguishable. Furthermore, it is well recognized that cytologic specimens from the kidney consisting of cells from tubules of various order, glomeruli and even pelvic epithelium are more heterogeneous and difficult to evaluate than specimens, for example, from the pancreas.

In 18 patients with renal carcinoma, no malignant cells were obtained. This could be due to missing the tumor, failed aspiration, or an incorrect evaluation by the cytologist.

Retroperitoneal and Miscellaneous Lesions

A small number of retroperitoneal (15) and miscellaneous (7) lesions underwent percutaneous fine needle biopsy using the same technique detailed above. All cases were verified by surgery or autopsy. Ten cases proved to be benign, and no false positives were recorded. In only five cases of malignant tumors did the aspirated material reveal malignant cells, and in one case,

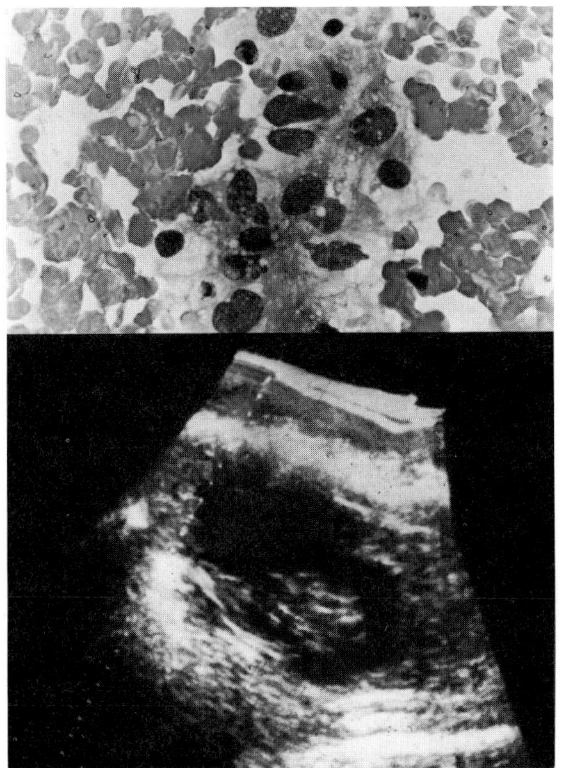

FIGURE 8. Solid tumor in the upper pole of a kidney. The cytologic specimen demonstrates malignant cells from the kidney.

TABLE 2. Kidney lesions—results of diagnosis by ultrasonically guided needle biopsy compared with final diagnosis.

			Cytological findings		
		Total	**Malignant Cells**	**No Malignant Cells**	**Insufficient Material**
Final Diagnosis	Malignant	141	119	18	4
	Benign	53	7	40	6
	Total	194	126	58	10

insufficient material was obtained. In six cases of obvious malignant tumors no malignant cells were aspirated.

These results are not very impressive, but are comparable to others, for fine needle aspiration from retroperitoneal tumors. In most cases it was quite obvious that the needle was in contact with the tumor mass; however, no malignant cells could be aspirated. The textures and consistencies of retroperitoneal tumors, including lymph node metastases, are often very hard. The type of needle and the technique used has probably not been optimal in these specific tumors.

Liver

Ultrasonically guided fine needle biopsy is indicated in primary liver tumors or metastatic lesions.[6] The patient should suspend respiration during the procedure to avoid trauma to the liver caused by motion. In liver metastases from an unknown primary tumor, a gross needle biopsy guided by ultrasound is most helpful in yielding a histological biopsy which may suggest the site of the primary tumor. Gross needle biopsy from the liver is routinely carried out with a Menghini or a Tru-Cut® needle. If desired, these needles can be introduced through the biopsy transducer if the adaptor is removed.

Hazards

At the Ultrasonic Laboratory, Herlev Hospital, approximately 2000 ultrasonically guided percutaneous punctures have been performed, including more than 500 from malignant lesions.

Fine Needle Biopsies

Complications demanding any kind of treatment such as surgery or transfusion have never occurred. The potential risk of spreading tumor cells is, of course, of the greatest importance when biopsy from a suspected malignant lesion is considered.[7, 8] Animal experiments seem to show that this problem is more of theoretical than of practical importance. In the present series of biopsied malignant tumors not a single case has shown local tumor growth, such as skin metastases, which would reasonably correlate with the fine needle aspiration biopsy procedure.

Hemorrhage is another potential risk of the procedure. Until now there has been no material published about bleeding following fine needle biopsy. This series contains two cases, where surgery after a biopsy procedure incidentally disclosed hematomas in relation to the site of the biopsy. One was a well-demarcated hematoma surrounding a lower pole kidney tumor, and one hematoma encircled an adenoma in the adrenal.

Infection, bile leakage or fistula formation have never been observed. In many cases the needle traverses the liver or gastrointestinal tract, apparently without any harm. It is worth remembering that suture needles for abdominal surgery are thicker than the 23-gauge needle used for the biopsy procedure. Pneumothorax occasionally follows ordinary liver biopsy, but has never occurred in connection with the fine needle biopsy.

Lumbar Needle Punctures

It is not known whether the use of a 1.2 mm (18-gauge) needle for puncture of malignant lesions increases the risk of seeding tumor cells. We have therefore omitted its use for the puncture of solid lesions. It has, however, been used in hundreds of other lesions almost without complication. One such complication occurred two months after the biopsy of a pancreatic pseudocyst, when an adjacent hematoma was disclosed at operation. Recently, a puncture of a gallbladder followed by contrast injection disclosed a large, unexpected stone in the common bile duct. Six hours later, the patient showed signs of a bile leak. At operation, when the stone was removed, 500 ml of bile was found in the peritoneum.

Summary

Under ultrasonic guidance it is possible to perform percutaneous punctures for diagnostic and therapeutic purposes with ease and great accuracy. The procedure, which in daily clinical work has proved to be of great value in the evaluation of a large number of abdominal lesions, carries a minimal risk.

References

1. Holm HH, Kristensen JK, Rasmussen SN, Northeved A, Barlebo H: Ultrasound as a guide in percutaneous puncture technique. Ultrasonics, 83–86, 1972.
2. Petersen JF, Cowan DF, Kristensen JK, Holm HH, Hancke S, Jensen F: Ultrasonically guided percutaneous nephrostomy. Radiology 119:429–431, 1976.
3. Hancke S, Holm HH, Kock F: Ultrasonically guided percutaneous fine needle biopsy of the pancreas. Surg Gyn Obstet 140:361–364, 1975.
4. Kristensen JK, Holm HH, Rasmussen SN, Barlebo H: Ultrasonically guided percutaneous puncture of renal masses. Scand J Urol Nephrol, 6, supplement 15:49, 1972.
5. Franszén S: Studier över värdet av punktionscytologi vid diagnostik av tumorsjukdomar. Thesis, Stockholm 1968.
6. Rasmussen SN, Holm HH, Kristensen JK, Barlebo H: Ultrasonically guided liver biopsy. Brit Med J 2:500–502, 1972.
7. Engzel V, Esposti PL, Rubio C, Sigurdson A, Zajcik J: Investigation of tumor spread in connection with aspiration biopsy. Acta Radiol 10:385–399, 1971.
8. von Schreeb T, Arner O, Skovsted G, Wikstad N: Renal adenocarcinoma: is there a risk of spreading tumor cells in diagnostic puncture?: Scan J Urol Nephrol 1:270–276, 1967.

CASE NO. 1

W. F. Sample and D. A. Sarti

Epigastic Mass in an Alcoholic

A 54 year-old Caucasian male with a long history of alcohol abuse entered the hospital complaining of upper abdominal mid-epigastric pain. On physical examination, an epigastric mass was palpated but could not be separated from the liver. Laboratory evaluation revealed a normal hematocrit, white blood count and differential. SGOT, SGPT and alkaline phosphatase were normal. A total serum bilirubin was 1.0 mg% and the serum amylase was only slightly elevated. A liver/spleen scan demonstrated a possible filling defect in the left lobe of the liver. A transverse gray-scale sonogram (Figure 1) and a transverse computed tomogram (Figure 2) through the region of the mass are provided.

Labelling key: R = left; gb = gallbladder; cd = common bile duct; p = pancreas; smv = superior mesenteric vein; sma = superior mesenteric artery; I = inferior vena cava; a = aorta; k = kidney; st = stomach; M = mass.

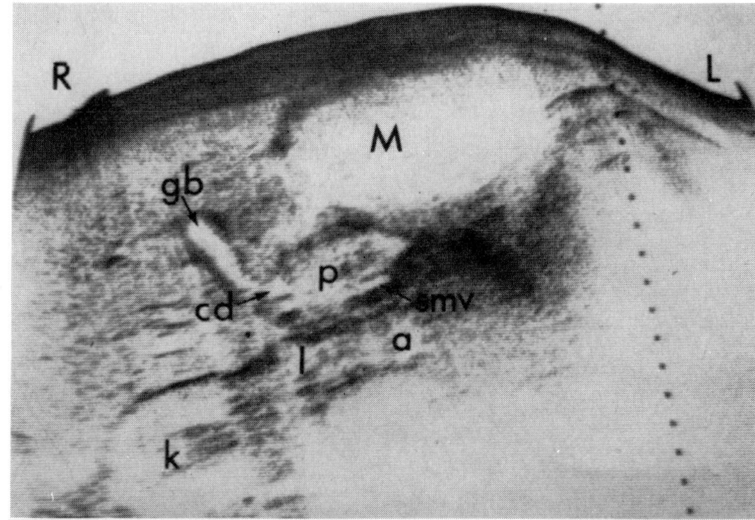

FIGURE 1

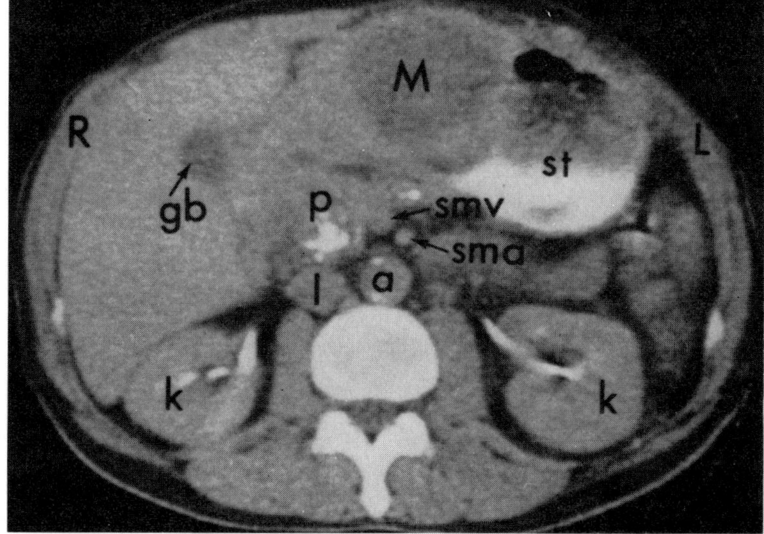

FIGURE 2

DISCUSSION

The transverse gray-scale sonogram demonstrates a thick-walled cystic mass which is apparently separated from the head of the pancreas. However, the visualized portion of the head of the pancreas demonstrates an abnormal texture with generalized decreased echogenicity and several areas of focal increased echogenicity. The common bile duct is towards the upper limits of normal in size. The computed tomogram confirms the thick-walled fluid nature of the mass as well as the suspected presence of calcification within the pancreas. Both studies demonstrate a cleavage plane between the mass and the left lobe of the liver, which is somewhat small in this patient, probably accounting for the questionable defect on the liver/spleen scan. On the ultrasonogram alone, it is uncertain whether the mass is arising from the pancreas or, conceivably, from the stomach or duodenum. Evaluation of the mass in a number of positions or following nasogastric tube evacuation of the stomach would be necessary to ensure that it was not gastric in origin. The computed tomogram, however, delineates the stomach by means of oral iodinated contrast, and thereby establishes its extragastric origin.

The findings on the combined study are compatible with the development of a pseudocyst in a patient with chronic pancreatitis. Although a cleavage plane between the mass and the pancreas is present, this should not prevent one from making this diagnosis. Pseudocysts frequently dissect through the tissue planes and end up a considerable distance from the pancreatic bed itself. Although a necrotic tumor, cystadenoma or cystadenocarcinoma of the pancreas could never be excluded on either of these studies, the simple nature of the fluid collection as well as the fairly smooth, thick wall would favor the diagnosis of an uncomplicated pseudocyst. The absence of strong reflective material within the cystic mass on the ultrasonogram, and the absence of air within the mass on the computed tomogram are against the diagnosis of a pancreatic abscess.

Final diagnosis: Chronic pancreatitis with pseudocyst formation.

REFERENCES

1. Conrad MR, Landay MJ, Khoury M. Pancreatic pseudocysts: unusual ultrasound features. Am J Roentgenol 130:265–268, 1978.
2. Gooding GAW. Pseudocyst of the pancreas with mediastinal extension: an ultrasonographic demonstration. J Clin Ultrasound 5:121–123, 1977.

CASE NO. 2

W. F. Sample and D. A. Sarti

Acute Abdominal Pain in a Young Female

A 30 year-old Caucasian female presented to the emergency room with acute upper abdominal pain, nausea and vomiting. Physical examination was unremarkable with the exception of epigastric tenderness on deep palpation. Routine laboratory evaluation revealed a normal white blood count, hematocrit, liver enzymes and urinalysis. Serum amylase was moderately elevated. Figures 1, 2, and 3 represent transverse gray-scale sonograms taken at the same level over a period of two minutes.
Labelling key: GB = gallbladder; K = right kidney; I = inferior vena cava; A = aorta; SMV = superior mesenteric vein.

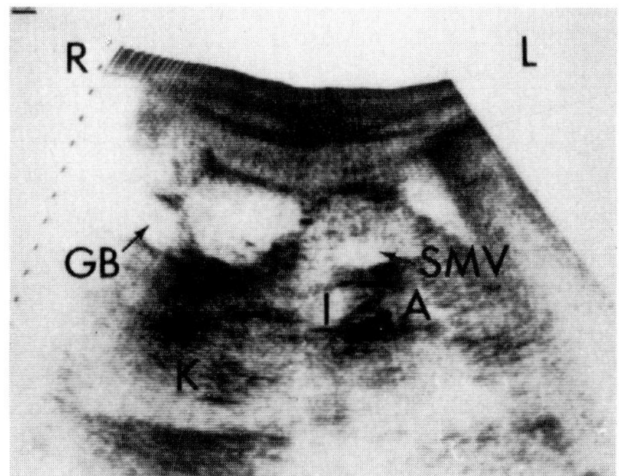

FIGURE 1

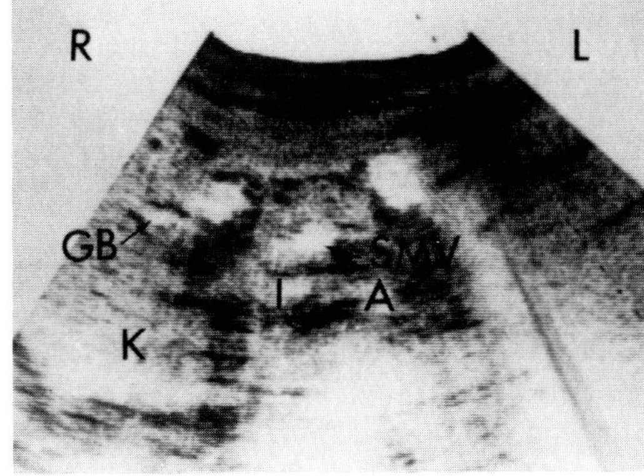

FIGURE 2

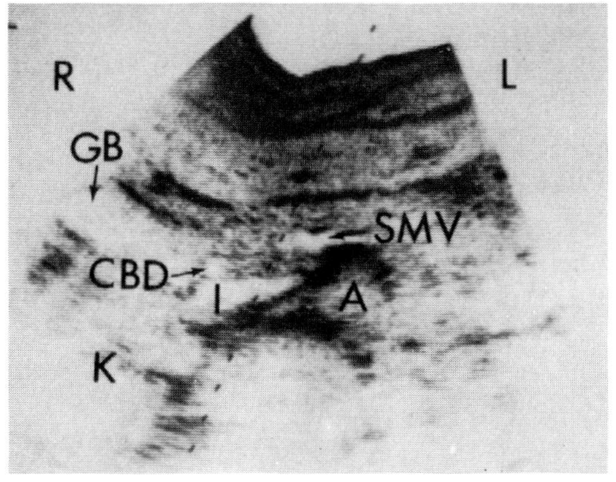

FIGURE 3

DISCUSSION

The transverse gray-scale sonogram shows the pancreas to be slightly enlarged, with a solid type of generalized decreased echogenicity. On the first sonogram (Figure 1) an irregular fluid area is noted between the gallbladder and the head of the pancreas. However, serial sonograms over a period of two minutes, demonstrate this fluid area to decrease in size and, finally, to disappear into the configuration of a gas pocket. Although the initial interpretation might have been a pancreatic pseudocyst, the changing nature of this fluid region should suggest dilated bowel. Adynamic type of ileus frequently accompanies acute pancreatitis, and is not always as easy to demonstrate as this case would suggest. Sometimes positional changes will show the passage of fluid within the bowel around the duodenal sweep or, as in other cases, nasogastric suction may be necessary to demonstrate the intraluminal source of the fluid. The stomach and duodenal sweep may have a variety of ultrasonic patterns depending upon whether the bowel is collapsed, fluid-filled or food-filled. Once these various patterns are learned, fewer mistakes in the differential diagnosis of upper abdominal masses will occur.

Final diagnosis: Acute pancreatitis with adynamic ileus.

REFERENCES

1. Sample WF. Techniques for improved delineation of normal anatomy of the upper abdomen and high retroperitoneum with gray scale ultrasound. Radiology 124:197–202, 1977.
2. Sokoloff J, Gosink BB, Leopold GR, Forsythe JR. Pitfalls in the echographic evaluation of pancreatic disease. J Clin Ultrasound 2:321–326, 1974.

CASE NO. 3 Alan Dembner

Abdominal Pain in an Elderly Male

A 69 year-old man presented with a chief complaint of intermittent episodes of abdominal pain. He had a previous history of nodular lymphoma which responded to radio- and chemotherapy. Physical examination and laboratory examinations were unremarkable. Upper GI series, barium enema, excretory urography and liver/spleen scans were normal. An abdominal ultrasound examination (Figures 1a and b) was performed to exclude the pancreas as an origin of the patient's pain. Key structures are labelled with numbers for the reader's participation. A special procedure was performed.

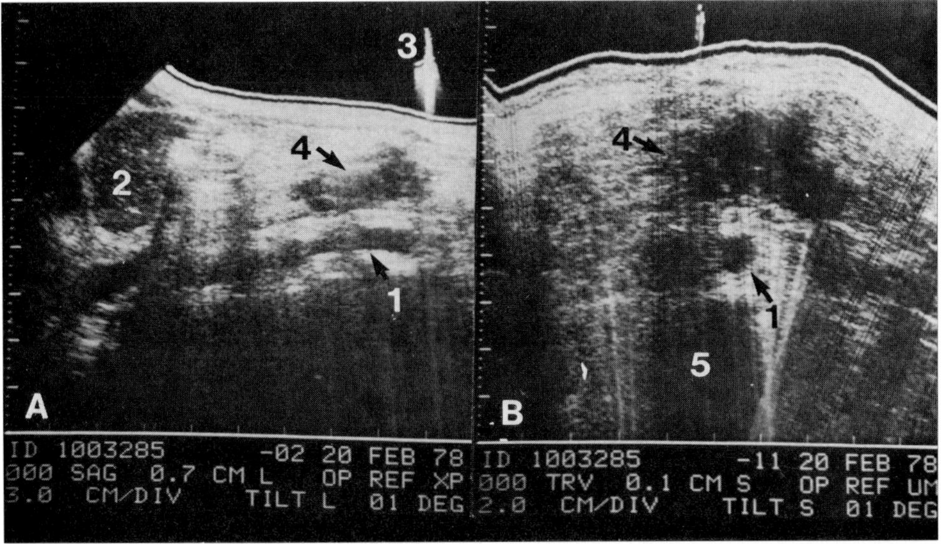

FIGURE 1

DISCUSSION

A sagittal section approximately 2 cm to the left of the midline (Figure 1a) demonstrates the aorta (1) and the left lobe of the liver (2), with a marker at the area of the umbilicus (3). There is a lobular, sonolucent mass (4) extending from the retroperitoneum to the mesenteric area. A transverse sonogram in the area of interest demonstrates a mass (4), aorta (1), and spine (5).

The mass was clearly below the pancreas and most likely represented a recurrent lymphoma. The special procedure performed was an ultrasonically guided, skinny-needle biopsy. Lymphocytes were obtained that correlated with the patient's previously diagnosed lymphoma. The patient was started on chemotherapy and thus avoided laparotomy.

Characteristically, lymphadenopathy presents as a very sonolucent, but lobular mass. It may efface the retroperitoneal great vessels, and enter into the mesentery and porta hepatis. Although it is sonolucent, there are internal echoes and poor through-transmission because of beam absorption. Ultrasonically guided biopsy of abdominal and retroperitoneal masses is a safe, quick and inexpensive way of diagnosing a multitude of lesions.

REFERENCES

1. Leopold GR: A review of retroperitoneal ultrasonography. J Clin Ultrasound 1: 75, 1973.
2. Brascho DJ, Durant JR, Green LE: The accuracy of retroperitoneal ultrasonography in Hodgkin's disease and non-Hodgkin's lymphoma. Radiology 125:485, 1977.
3. Holm HH, Pedersen FR, Kristensen JK, Rasmussen SN, Hancke S, Jensen F: Ultrasonically guided percutaneous puncture. Radiology Clinics of North America 8:493, 1975.

CASE NO. 4 Alan Dembner

Melanoma and Liver–Spleen Defect

A 46 year-old female who underwent a hysterectomy for uncontrollable vaginal bleeding had an incidental "nevus" removed from her thigh at the time of surgery. This skin lesion was histologically a grade 3 melanoma. Work-up of the lesion included a liver/spleen scan (Figure 1) which showed a defect in the liver. An abdominal ultrasound examination (Figure 2) was performed; key structures are labelled with numbers for the reader's participation. A special procedure was performed.

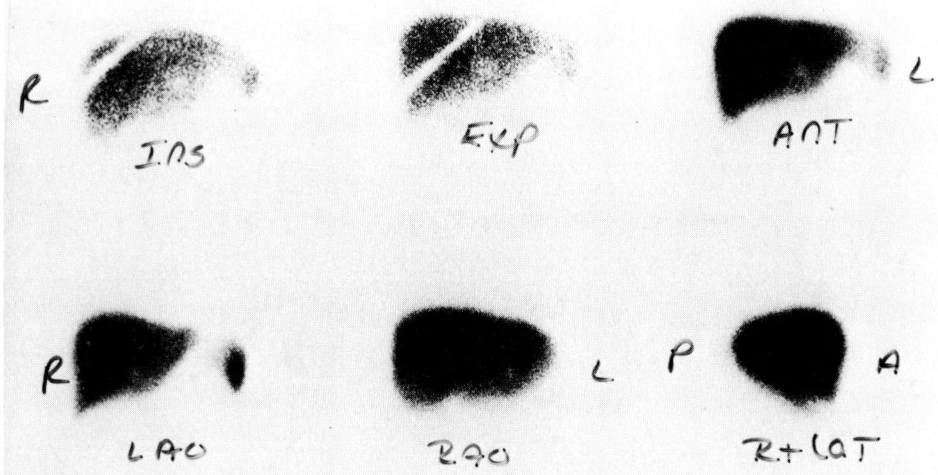

FIGURE 1

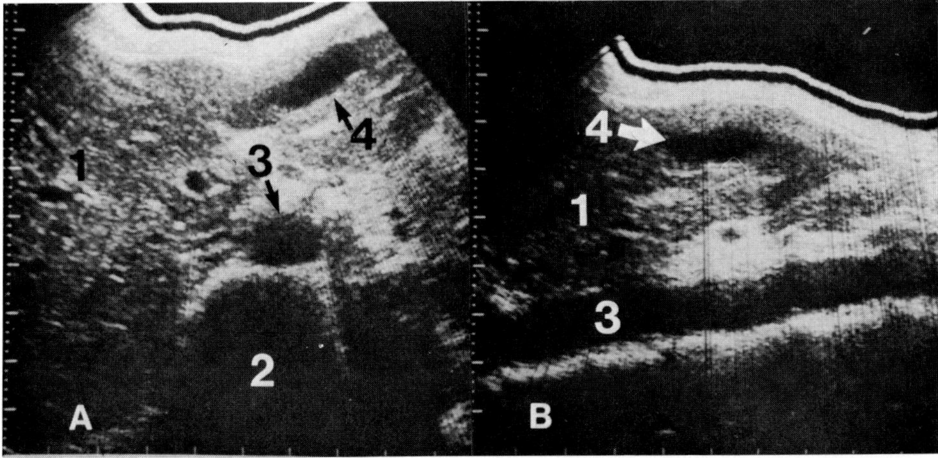

FIGURE 2

DISCUSSION

A transverse sonogram (Figure 2a) through the patient's liver (1) demonstrates the spine (2), aorta (3), and a fairly sonolucent lesion (4). The lesion, however, has some internal echoes, and the possibility of a metastatic lesion must be differentiated from an incidental cyst. A sagittal scan (Figure 2b) through the aorta (3) also demonstrates the mass (4) in the liver (1).

Gray-scale ultrasonography is an excellent way of defining lesions seen on radionuclide scans of the liver. It can differentiate prominent gallbladder and renal fossae, large vessels and dilated ducts from metastases, and can usually differentiate solid from cystic lesions. In this case, because of the patient's history and the suspicious nature of the lesion, an ultrasonographically guided aspiration biopsy was performed. Clear fluid was obtained and a post-aspiration scan (Figure 3) no longer demonstrated the lesion.

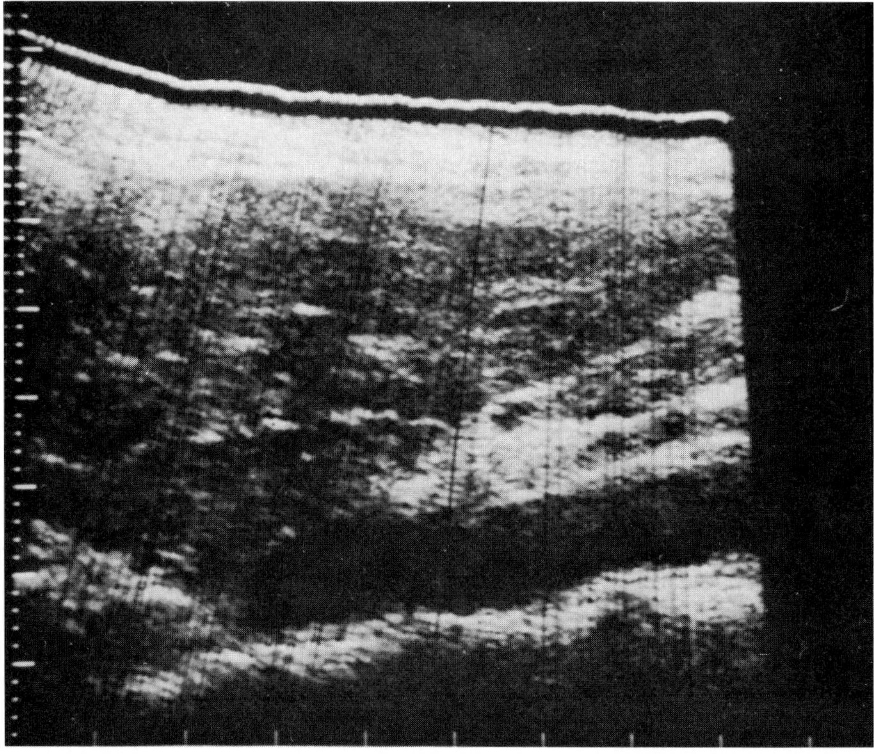

FIGURE 3

REFERENCES

1. Goldberg BD, Pollack HH: Ultrasonic aspiration biopsy techniques. J Clin Ultrasound 4:141, 1976.
2. Taylor KJW, Sullivan D, Rosenfield AT, Gottschalk A: Grey-scale ultrasound and isotope scanning: complementary techniques for imaging the liver. Am J Roentgenol 128:277, 1977.
3. Wellwood JM, Madara J, Cady B, Haggitt RC: Large interhepatic cysts and pseudocysts: pitfalls in diagnosis and treatment. Am J Surg 135:57, 1977.

CASE NO. 5 William Steel

Right Upper Quadrant Pain in an Elderly Male

A 70 year-old white male was admitted with fever, pain and rebound tenderness in the right upper quadrant. The temperature was 102° F. Leukocytosis and a shift to the left were noted. An ultrasound examination in the paramedian plane 7 cm to the right of the midline is shown in Figure 1. A radiologic procedure for confirmation was performed and the patient taken to surgery.

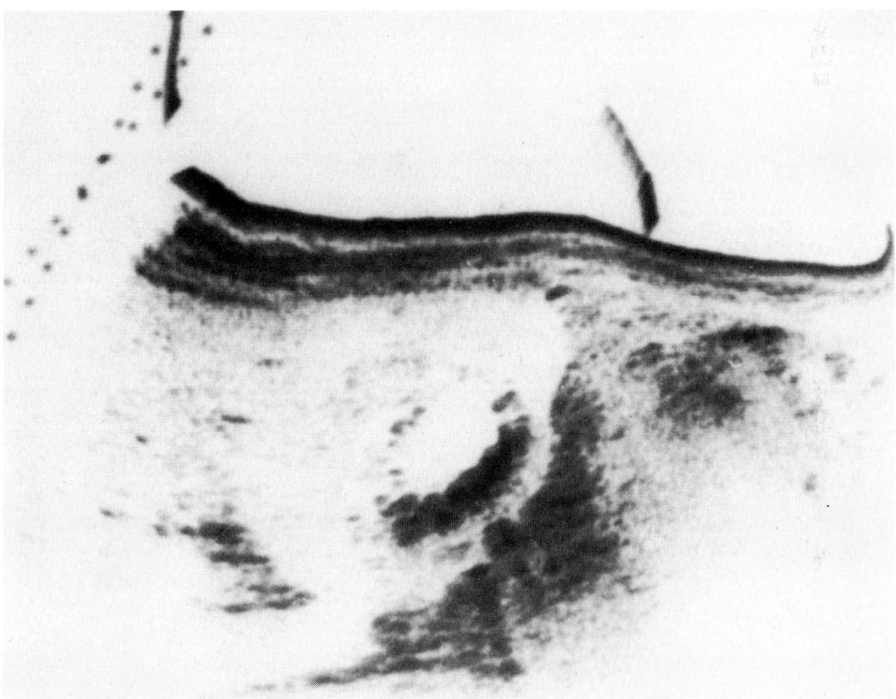

FIGURE 1. Paramedian ultrasonogram 7 cm to the right of the midline, through the region of the gallbladder.

DISCUSSION

A STAT intravenous cholangiogram (IVC) showed very poor concentration but essentially normal appearance of the common bile duct with no visualization of the gallbladder.

At surgery, a leaking, gangrenous gallbladder was found which contained many small gallstones. Cholecystostomy was performed.

The diagnosis was suggested on the ultrasonogram. Ill-defined shadowing is seen from opacities within the gallbladder, the gallbladder walls are thick, and there is a relatively echo-free area around the gallbladder (Figure 2, arrowed). This suggests the presence of gallstones and perforation of the gallbladder with the formation of a pericholecystic abscess.

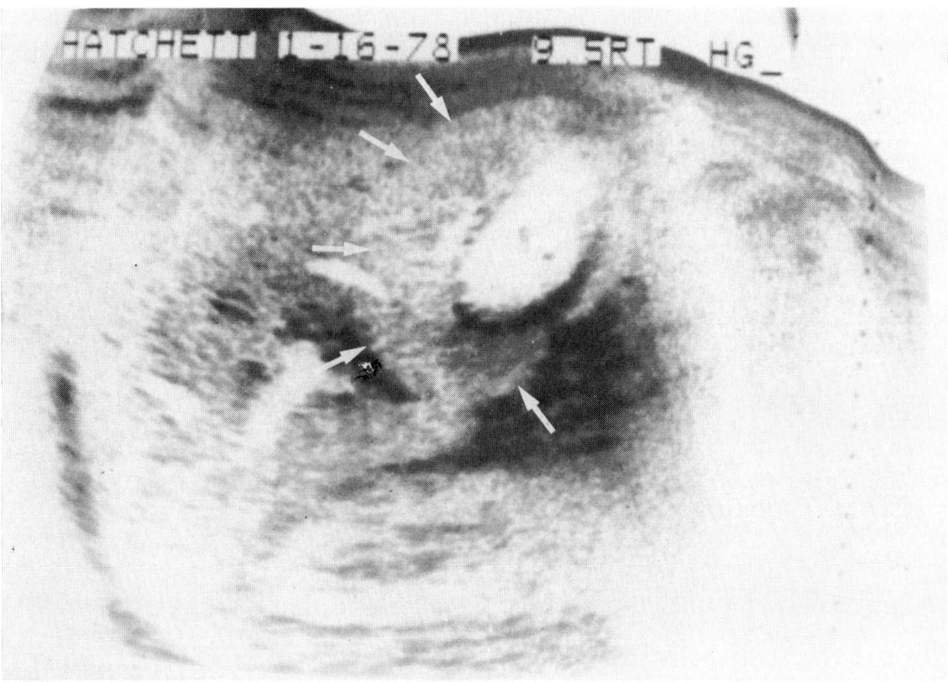

FIGURE 2. Paramedian ultrasonogram 9.5 cm to the right of the midline, showing the gallbladder lumen with thick walls. Shadowing from the opacities within the gallbladder is better seen in Figure 1. Notice that the gallbladder is surrounded by a relatively echo-free zone (arrowed). These appearances are consistent with perforation of the gallbladder and formation of a pericholecystic abscess.

CASE NO. 6 William Steel

Epigastic Pain in a Young Female

A 29 year-old black female was admitted with epigastric pain of four days duration prior to admission. The patient had a history of pancreatitis and alcohol abuse. She was referred for ultrasound of the gallbladder.

A transverse (Figure 1) and longitudinal (Figure 2) scan of the epigastric region are shown.

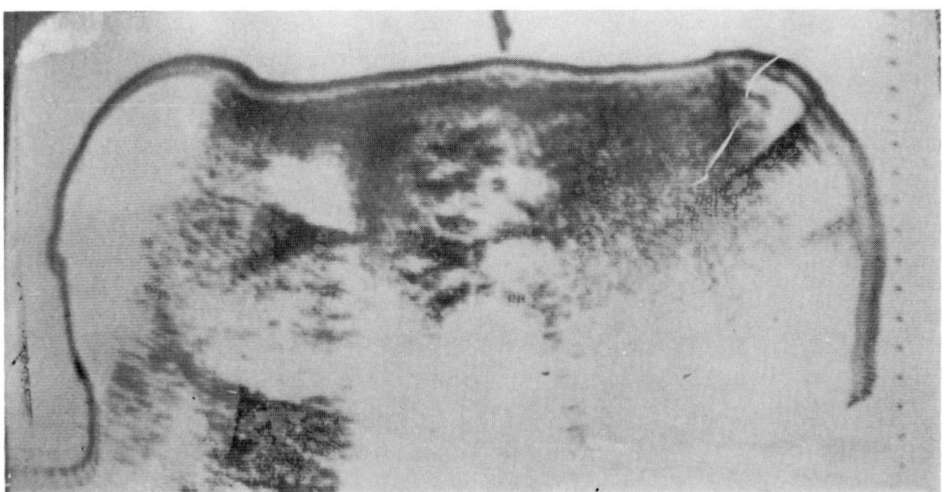

FIGURE 1. Transverse ultrasonogram at a level immediately below the xiphisternum.

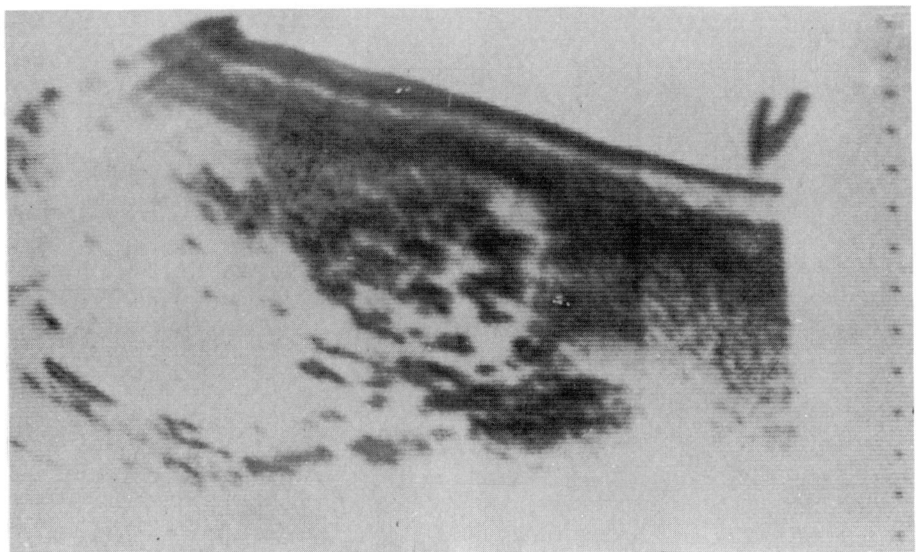

FIGURE 2. Paramedian ultrasonogram 3 cm to the right of the midline, through the region of the head of the pancreas.

DISCUSSION

The ultrasound appearances are consistent with chronic calcific pancreatitis with an acute exacerbation. The gallbladder is normal on scans. The mass in the region of the pancreas represents enlargement of the gland, with strong punctate echoes due to areas of calcification. These are well demonstrated on the scans, in contrast to the edematous swelling of the rest of the gland around these areas of calcification.

An upper gastrointestinal barium examination (Figure 3) shows only modest widening of sweep, but there is severe duodenitis (arrowed). On a follow-up ultrasound scan (Figure 4) the gland is reduced in size, the calcifications are aggregated and demonstrate shadowing with poor through transmission, rendering it more difficult to outline the gland in the quiescent stage.

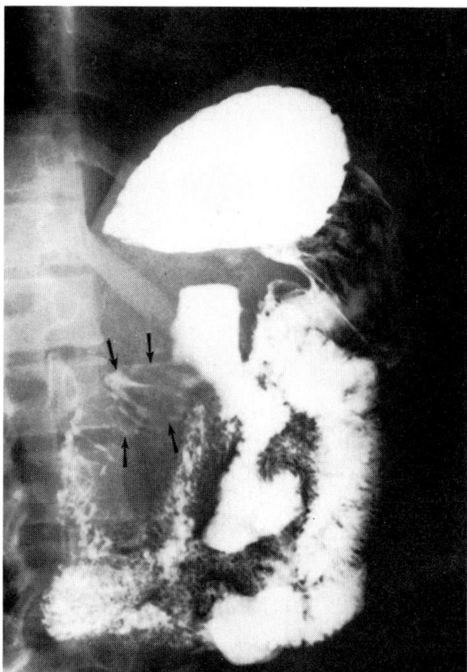

FIGURE 3. Upper gastrointestinal barium examination showing abnormal mucosal pattern in the duodenum, consistent with duodenitis (arrowed).

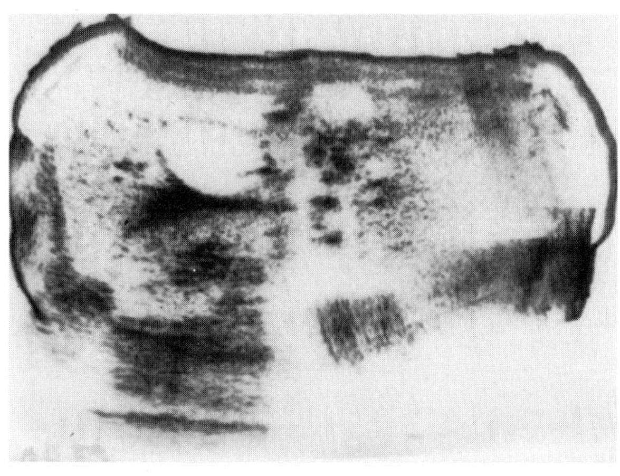

FIGURE 4. Transverse ultrasonogram (compare with Figure 1). Note that the pancreas (arrowed) is smaller than on the previous examination and the gland is less well delineated.

CASE NO. 7 D. O. Cosgrove

Melanoma and Liver–Spleen Defect

A 47 year-old farmer's wife from the West of England had had a malignant melanoma excised from her left leg 2 years previously. In the past 3 months she had noticed a swelling in the left groin, had begun to lose weight, with anorexia and, more recently, nausea and vomiting. She was exposed to both sheep and dogs and Echinococcus is endemic, though uncommon, in the remoter parts of England.

On examination she was obviously unwell and dehydrated, with evident recent weight loss. The leg scar was well-healed with no local recurrence, but the inguinal nodes were obviously involved and she had marked hepatomegaly. Initial investigations revealed a normochromic anemia with moderate elevation of liver enzymes. Bilirubin was normal, but urinary melanogens were raised. Screening for further metastatic disease resulted in normal chest and plain abdominal X-ray films. Bone scanning and marrow aspiration were also normal. The liver scan revealed a large filling defect in the right lobe. Ultrasound scans at presentation are shown in Figures 1, 2 and 3. Figure 4 is a section through the same plane as Figure 3, taken 3 weeks later. In the interim the patient had been treated with high dose melphelan, but clinically she had deteriorated.

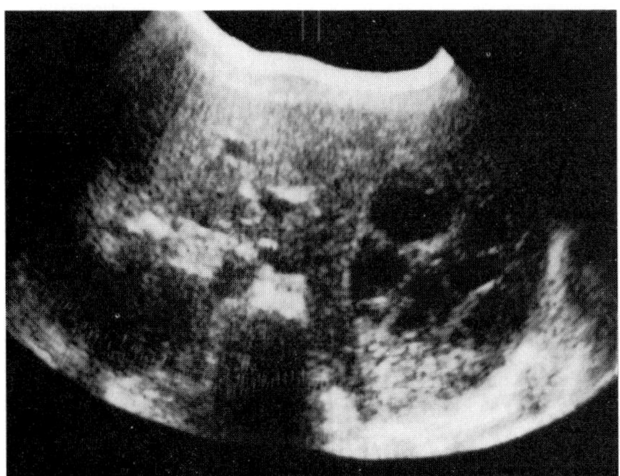

FIGURE 1. Transverse section in the epigastrium.

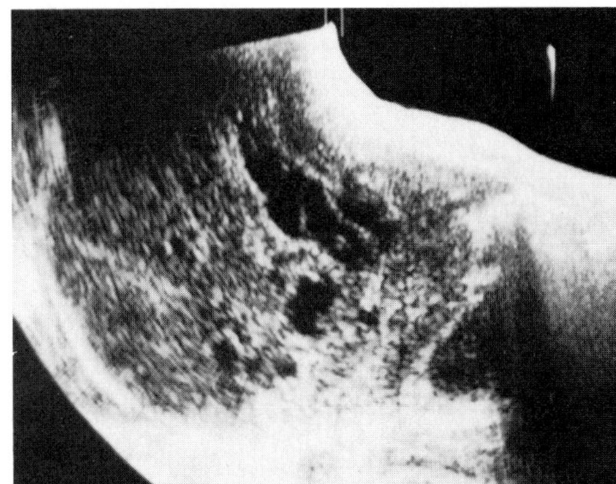

FIGURE 2. Sagittal section 4 cm to the right of midline.

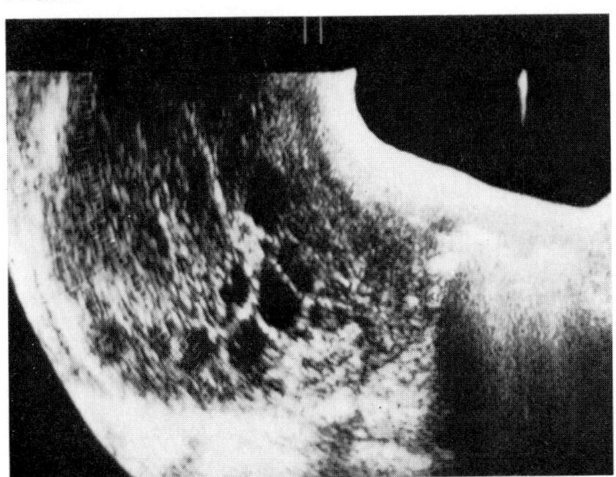

FIGURE 3. Sagittal section 8 cm to the right of midline.

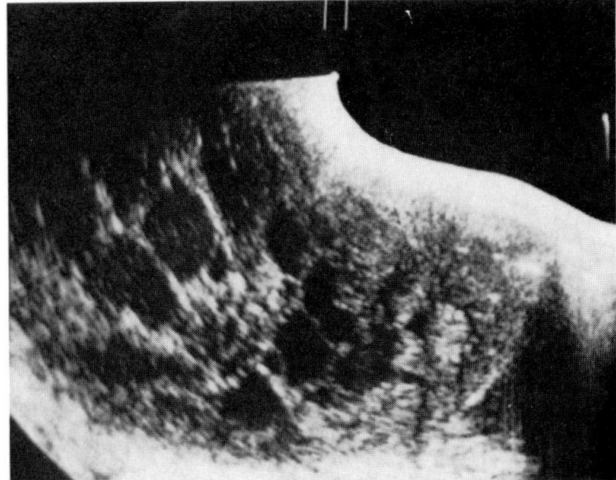

FIGURE 4. Repeat sagittal section 8 cm to the right of midline after three weeks.

DISCUSSION

The ultrasonograms show a large, complex, abnormal region in the posterior portion of the right lobe of the liver. It consists of a number of contiguous rounded 0.5 – 2.0 cm regions of low or absent reflectivity, some of which show increased through transmission (Figures 5 – 7). The left lobe is normal. The portion of kidney seen is normal and this was confirmed on prone scanning of the kidneys. Three weeks later the mass has enlarged and there has been further reduction in the echo levels of its components (Figure 8).

At initial presentation the differential diagnosis on ultrasound was considered to rest between hydatid disease and a complex of partially necrotic metastases. An abscess complex seemed unlikely on clinical grounds. Polycystic hepatic disease was considered, but this is characteristically a generalized liver disease and about half of these cases have renal involvement also (although only about a third of renal cases have associated hepatic involvement). Disturbance of liver enzymes is not a feature of polycystic disease. A congenital hamartomatous vascular lesion (hemangioma) could produce this appearance, but again without the enzyme release, and the hepatomegaly produced would have excited interest at her initial presentation with the cutaneous melanoma.

Hydatid liver disease is predominantly right-sided and, when mature, the enlarging daughter cysts within the primary hydatid produce this sort of "bunch of cysts" appearance. Debris (hydatid sand) within the cyst can give rise to internal echoes. Hydatid cysts are commonly asymptomatic, apart from discomfort due to the bulk of the lesion. Solitary hydatid cysts also occur and these are indistinguishable from unilocular benign cysts. The history of exposure to sheep and dogs is in favor of this diagnosis. Necrotic metastases can be cystic, usually with ragged walls, and are sometimes, but not always, tender. Usually there are also solid metastases in other parts of the liver. Metastases from melanoma are always low in echo content and not infrequently necrotic. However, a group of deposits localized to one part of the liver is an unusual distribution. Partly to give the patient the benefit of the doubt the first ultrasound examination was reported as "probably hydatid cyst, possibly necrotic deposit — please refer back for a repeat examination." Negative serology for echinococcus, a normal liver echogram in her husband and the rapid growth of the lesion over the next 3 weeks, with the appearance of further necrotic lesions, pointed strongly to a malignant etiology and this proved to be the diagnosis at autopsy a month later, when massive involvement of the right lobe of the liver by necrotic melanoma was found.

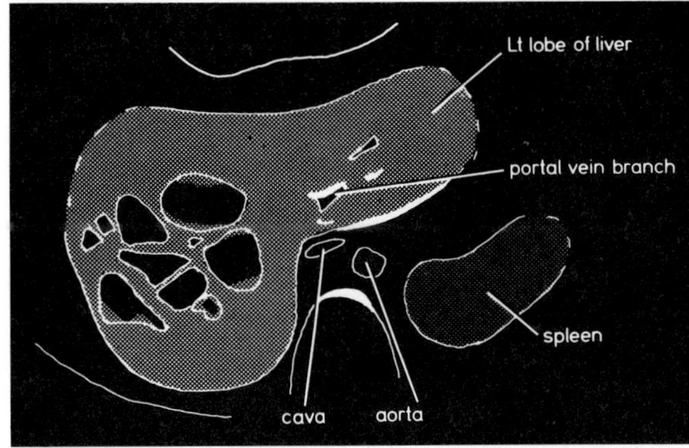

FIGURE 5. Schematic diagram of ultrasound scan shown in Figure 1.

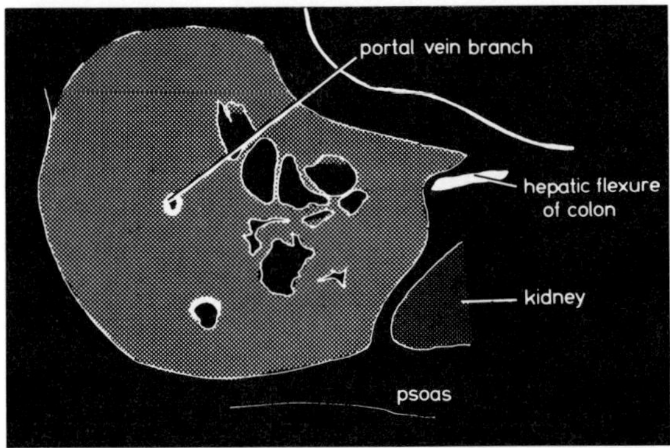

FIGURE 6. Schematic diagram of ultrasound scan shown in Figure 2.

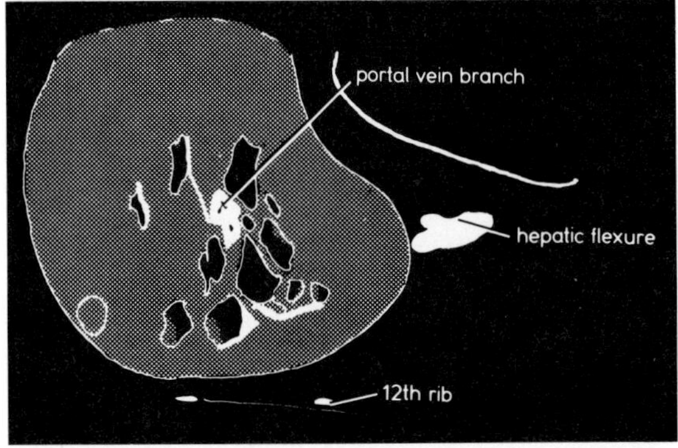

FIGURE 7. Schematic diagram of ultrasound scan shown in Figure 3.

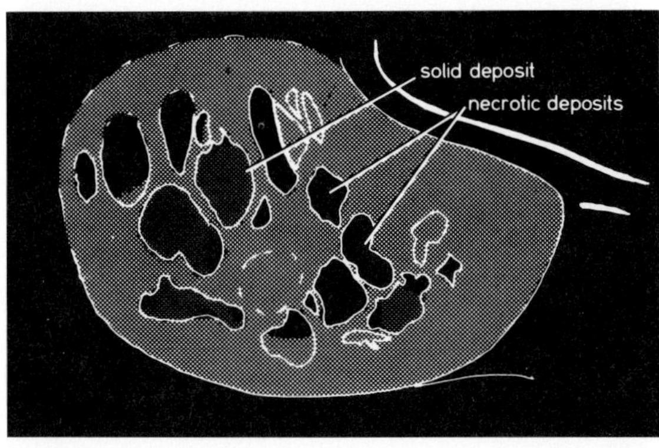

FIGURE 8. Schematic diagram of ultrasound scan shown in Figure 4.

CASE NO. 8 D. O. Cosgrove

Pulsatile Abdominal Mass in an Elderly Male

A 63 year-old man presented with malaise, weight loss and vague abdominal pain. On examination he looked unwell and had pale mucosae. There was a mild abdominal mass which was pulsatile, but it was difficult to be sure whether the pulsation was transmitted or intrinsic. Otherwise the abdomen was normal. On plain abdominal X-ray there was aortic calcification. There was a normochromic anemia and mild elevation of liver enzymes, including the gamma glutamyl transaminase.

Ultrasound examination of the aorta is shown in Figure 1. There were abnormalities in the liver, as shown in Figures 2 and 3. The spleen and kidneys were normal, but the preaortic area was obscured by gas.

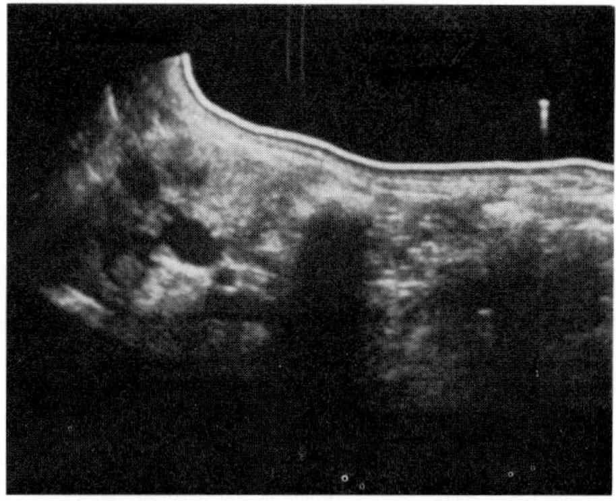

FIGURE 2. Sagittal section 2 cm to the right of midline.

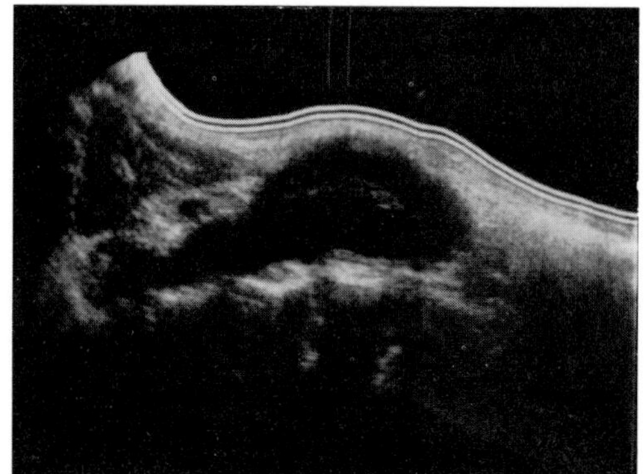

FIGURE 1. Sagittal section in the midline.

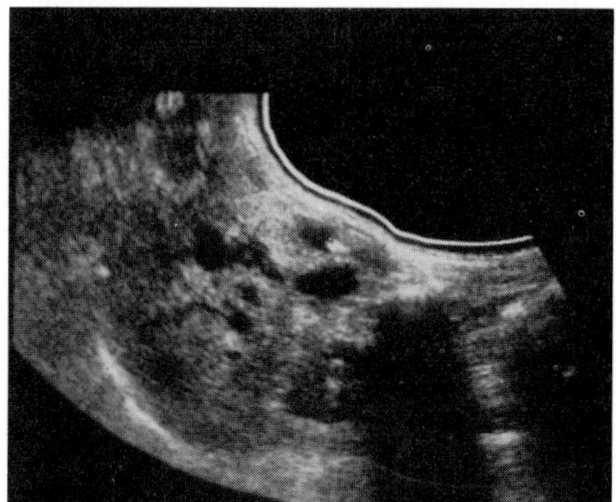

FIGURE 3. Sagittal section 6 cm to the right of midline.

DISCUSSION

Figure 1 shows a large fusiform aneurysm containing thrombus without evidence of leakage. Apart from the aneurysm, the ultrasonograms (Figures 2 and 3) show multiple, rounded and irregular regions of reduced reflectivity scattered through the enlarged liver. Some show increased through transmission and are fluid-filled, and some have no detectable internal echo. Others display a target pattern of concentric alternating rings of high and low reflectivity. Their walls are irregular, at least in part, and several show connections with vascular structure.

The pattern was interpreted as being due to multiple metastases, some necrotic. The possibility that this was polycystic disease was discounted because of the irregular ill-defined walls and the presence of internal echoes. In addition there were no renal cysts, which are a common association. The vessels were thought to be tumor-feeding vessels. Ultrasonically guided liver biopsy was recommended but, since the patient had been referred from another hospital, this was logistically difficult and he went to laparotomy. The aneurysm was confirmed and the liver was found to contain numerous deposits, many necrotic. A carcinoma of the body of the pancreas was the primary site. The patient died in the postoperative period.

Ultrasonic diagnosis of liver metastases over about 2 cm in diameter is highly reliable. They usually appear as more or less rounded masses of low reflectivity, and offer attenuation which is the same as normal liver. Highly reflective metastases are not uncommon, occurring in larger lesions especially of urogenital and gastrointestinal tract primaries, but are very uncommon in sarcomas, lymphomas and melanomas. Necrotic metastases pose a difficult ultrasonic problem because they may simulate cysts, abscesses and hemangiomas. They may be associated with acute inflammation (fever, leukocytosis and tenderness). They usually have ill-defined shaggy walls, as in this example, unlike cysts, which have smooth clear margins. Feeding vessels can often be identified with hemangiomata but may also occur in relation to tumors. Pulse Doppler and real-time devices are likely to be helpful modalities in these difficult problems. Isotope dynamic studies can help detect hemangiomas. Unfortunately gallium scans are not useful, since both abscesses and tumors may concentrate the isotope. Target lesions with concentric rings of altering bands of reflectivity seem to be a specific pattern seen only in malignant deposits.

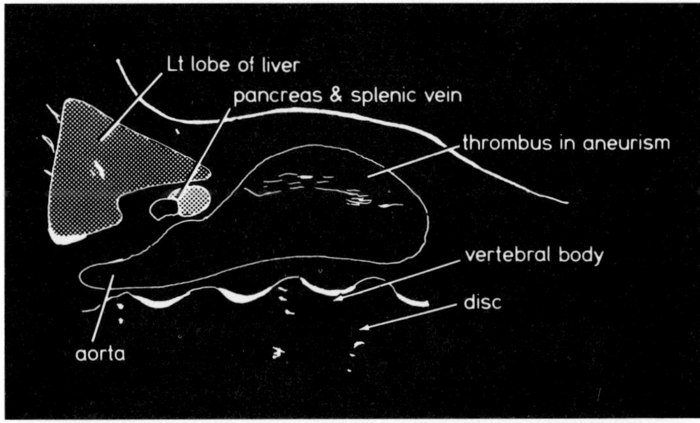

FIGURE 4

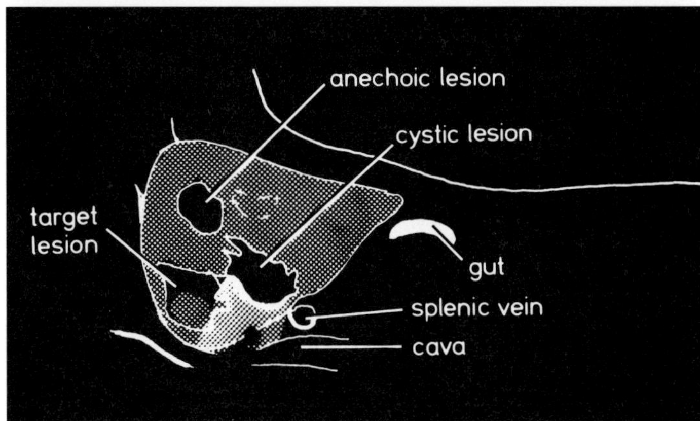

FIGURE 5

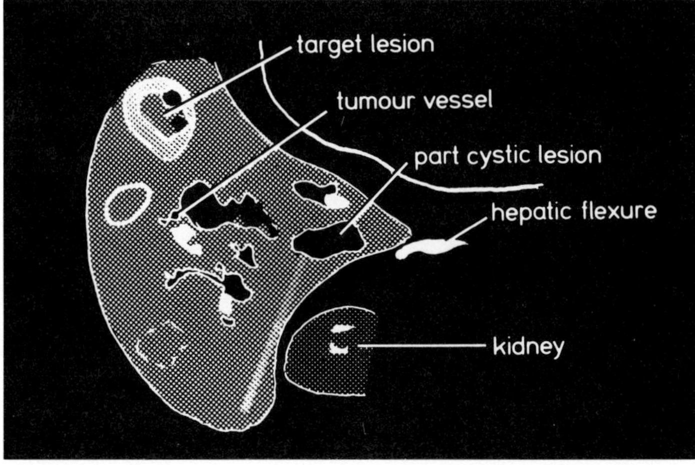

FIGURE 6

FIGURES 4, 5 and 6. Schematic diagrams of ultrasonograms shown in Figures 1, 2, and 3. Note the increased through transmission beyond the cystic and part cystic lesions in Figures 5 and 6. A target lesion usually shows as a reflective center with a poorly reflective rim, as in Figure 5. The reverse pattern, as in Figure 6, may also be seen.

CASE NO. 9 D. O. Cosgrove

Fever and Weight Loss in an Egyptain Male

A 46 year-old Arab male was referred from Egypt for investigation of malaise with intermittent fevers and weight loss over the last 6 – 12 months. Occult neoplasia was suspected although no obvious primary site was apparent. Apart from emaciation, clinical examination revealed only a vague epigastric resistance and a just palpable spleen, but the biochemical profile showed slight elevation of serum alkaline phosphatase with normal amino transferases and bilirubin. There was eosinophilia with a normal total white blood count, and there was a moderate hypochromic anemia with low serum iron and an elevated binding capacity. Occult malignancy with liver metastases indeed seemed likely and he was referred for ultrasonic scanning.

Two of the tomograms of his liver examination are shown in Figures 1 and 2, together with a transverse section through a normal liver for comparison (Figure 3). Scans of the kidneys and pelvis were unremarkable, but the spleen was slightly enlarged with a uniform echo pattern.

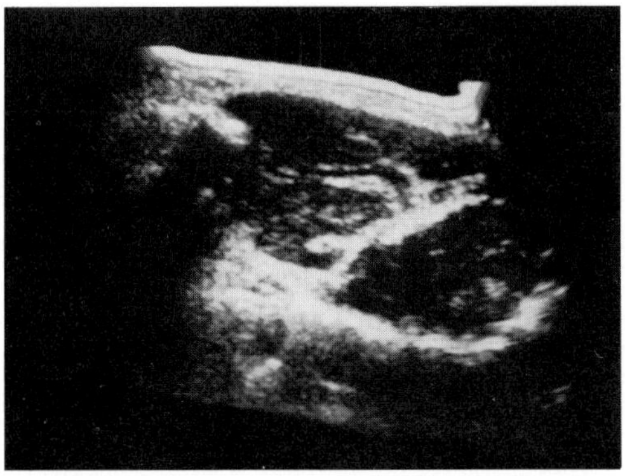

FIGURE 1. Epigastric transverse section.

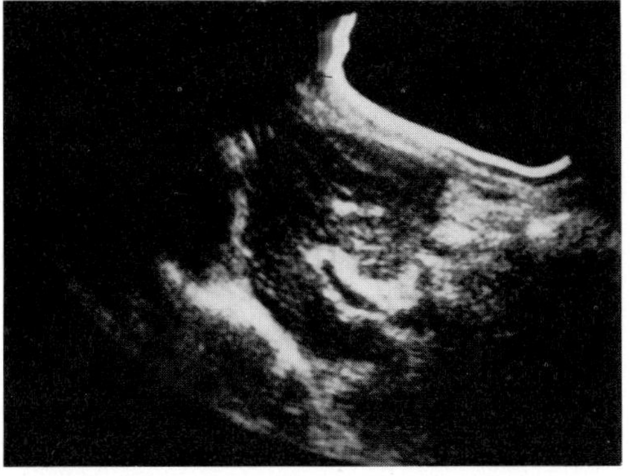

FIGURE 2. Sagittal section of the upper abdomen 1 cm to the right of the midline.

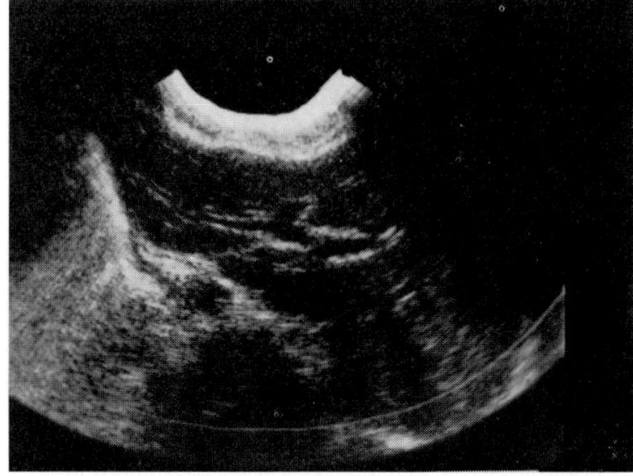

FIGURE 3. Epigastric transverse section of a normal subject using the same instrument settings as for Figures 1 and 2.

DISCUSSION

The ultrasound scans show enlargement of the left lobe of the liver, and a highly reflective cuff of tissue outlining vessels which converge to the porta hepatis. They are the portal vein and branches rather than dilated biliary vessels, which are beaded and parallel to the portal system. Indeed, rather than the increased sound transmission seen in gross biliary dilatation, these vessels are highly attenuating as judged by the shadowing produced over the liver, beyond the vein. The appearance suggests periportal fibrosis, and is that of pipe-stem cirrhosis.

The diagnosis of chronic schistosomiasis was supported by a positive schistosomal antibody titre. No trematode ova were recovered, but fecal occult bloods were positive. Predominant enlargement of the left lobe is common and an unexplained feature in this condition. Also characteristic is the excellent preservation of liver function in the face of disturbance of liver architecture. Ascites is a late finding and, even following bleeding from esophageal varices, decompensation is unusual.

On ultrasound the differential diagnosis includes other causes of hepatic fibrosis and of prominent vascular systems. In the common varieties of cirrhosis (portal and postnecrotic) the extent of fibrosis is very variable and is not closely correlated with the degree of hepatic decompensation. When prominent, the fibrosis produces the classic ultrasound pattern of high-level echoes accompanied by high attenuation. It is a diffuse process, usually affecting the liver uniformly, apart from the large regenerating nodules sometimes seen. In secondary biliary cirrhosis the same situation prevails, but with a variable degree of prominence of biliary vessels in addition. Congenital hepatic fibrosis is another diffuse process, and scarring following abscesses, congenital syphilis and trauma (surgical or accidental) though focal, is not specifically periportal. Fibrosis of periportal distribution may occur after chronic vinyl chloride exposure, but is milder than in schistosomiasis and may be complicated by angiosarcoma formation. Periportal cellular infiltration occurs in some cases of viral hepatitis, but produces only mild cuffing of the vessels on ultrasound.

Prominent hepatic veins are seen in right heart failure; these veins converge towards the inferior vena cava, and are thin-walled, tending to a sinusoidal rather than a true venous structure.

High reflectivity and attenuation can be associated with biliary vessels, most importantly in sclerosing cholangitis. In this condition, the beaded appearance of duct dilatation is exaggerated to produce a series of lacunae of bile, the intervening nipped-off zones being fibrosed and often casting shadows.

Further reading

TS Chen, PS Chen Essential Hepatology, Butterworth Company, Massachusetts, 1977, page 303.

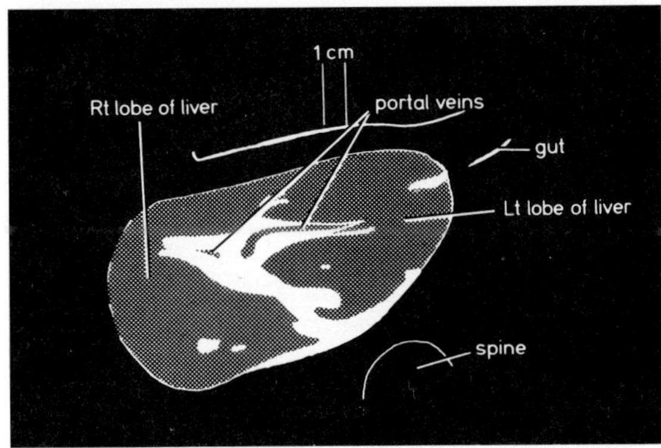

FIGURE 4. Epigastric transverse section—schematic diagram of ultrasound scan shown in Figure 1.

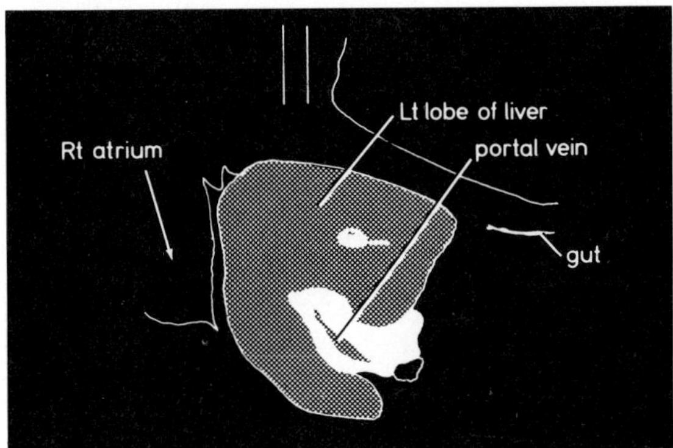

FIGURE 5. Upper abdominal surgical section 1 cm to the right of the midline—schematic diagram of ultrasound scan shown in Figure 2.

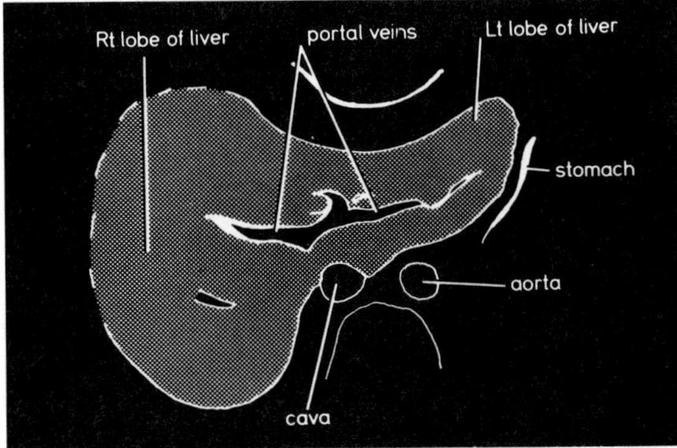

FIGURE 6. Epigastric transverse section in a normal subject—schematic diagram of ultrasound scan shown in Figure 3.

Index